THE ULTIMATE VIOLATION

THE ULTIMATE VIOLATION

VIOLATION

A Warning to All

KURTESS LIEF SCONE

iUniverse, Inc.
Bloomington

The Ultimate Violation
A Warning to All

Copyright © 2012 by Kurtess Lief Scone.

All rights reserved. No part of this book may be used or reproduced by any means, graphic, electronic, or mechanical, including photocopying, recording, taping or by any information storage retrieval system without the written permission of the publisher except in the case of brief quotations embodied in critical articles and reviews.

iUniverse books may be ordered through booksellers or by contacting:

iUniverse
1663 Liberty Drive
Bloomington, IN 47403
www.iuniverse.com
1-800-Authors (1-800-288-4677)

Because of the dynamic nature of the Internet, any web addresses or links contained in this book may have changed since publication and may no longer be valid. The views expressed in this work are solely those of the author and do not necessarily reflect the views of the publisher, and the publisher hereby disclaims any responsibility for them.

Any people depicted in stock imagery provided by Thinkstock are models, and such images are being used for illustrative purposes only.
Certain stock imagery © Thinkstock.

ISBN: 978-1-4759-0704-9 (sc)
ISBN: 978-1-4759-0705-6 (hc)
ISBN: 978-1-4759-0706-3 (ebk)

Library of Congress Control Number: 2012905564

Printed in the United States of America

iUniverse rev. date: 06/21/2012

CONTENTS

Author's Note ix

Precious Things xi

Introduction xv

Cosmetic Surgery Can Be Horrifying 1

The Double Mirror 6

My Adolescent Years 31

From Adolescence to Adulthood 50

The Adult Years 80

The Encounter 133

Trapped by a Psycho Doctor 168

Advice to the Reader 263

Postscript: To-Do List 265

Food for Thought 267

For the love of money is the root of all kinds of evil,
for which some have strayed from the faith in their greediness,
and pierced themselves
through with many sorrows.
1 Tim. 6:10

AUTHOR'S NOTE

The author has changed the names of most of the people and modified identifying features in some places of the other individuals in order to preserve their anonymity. The goal in all cases was to protect people's privacy without damaging the integrity of the story. The story is based on actual events.

PRECIOUS THINGS

There are precious things in life that we hold so dear that no one should ever take them from us. If they do, it can rob us of our dignity and leave us feeling violated and alone. When these precious things or possessions are taken from us in a careless or malicious manner, it can cause us to feel stripped and ripped off of their true value and our self-worth.

Special thanks to the,
"Hearst Communications, Inc./ Hearst Newspapers, LLC/Seattlepi.com."

I would like to give special credit to my sister Marlie and to my friend Bud for their contributions in making this book a great read for all people everywhere. Whether you are potentially interested in having cosmetic surgery in the near future, have had cosmetic surgery, or have had a botched surgery, you will want to read *The Ultimate Violation*.

INTRODUCTION

The following book by Kurtess Lief Scone is based on a true story. Some names have been changed to protect the guilty and the innocent. The events that negatively impacted my life were a slow, painful process that I endured for years. It took many more years to completely figure out everything that Dr. Cutter had mentally and cosmetically done to me.

My factual account is for every potential cosmetic consumer who desires to find the right cosmetic surgeon for himself or herself. The information in this book provides all the necessary tools and strategies about how to avoid the pitfalls of finding the wrong doctor. Without this information, you could sadly end up a victim of a cosmetic surgeon's interests in adding you to his files.

I would like to save the reader from ever being victimized by an uncaring, malicious medical predator. I would be extremely pleased to know that I was able to help even one person, and I hope that my book will educate millions. I would like to equip the reader on how to escape the clutches of being victimized by a medical doctor who cares more about professionally gaining your financial and cosmetic business than he or she does about your individual cosmetic interests.

Cosmetic Surgery Can Be Horrifying

In the right hands, cosmetic or plastic surgery can become an art of beauty and a tremendous self-esteem enhancement for a person's life. In the wrong hands, cosmetic surgery can literally become a powerful force to destroy one's self-esteem and any trace of confidence a person may have in the very core of his or her soul.

In the pursuit of finding the right cosmetic or plastic surgeon for myself, I happened to meet up with a cosmetic surgeon who, I came to realize, cared more about gaining my cosmetic and financial business than he cared about my cosmetic interests and desires. I only wish now that I had properly done my homework before I ever made an appointment to see the cosmetic surgeon who I came to realize was an opportunist predator.

Instead of having my self-esteem and self-image soaring with golden opportunities for the future, I was continuously obsessing about what had happened to me postsurgery and why any medical doctor would do what this cosmetic surgeon had done to me. I strongly hope that the reader of my book will never have to go through the devastating experiences that I have suffered in life. I never should have become the victim of cosmetic surgery.

Looking back upon the way the cosmetic doctor dealt with me, I can understand now that he was allowing me to come to my own conclusion that he could fulfill my cosmetic dreams for my facial features. After having the cosmetic doctor build up my confidence upon our initial consultation, things began to deteriorate during my second and third consultation. I recognize it now, but I didn't at the time of our consultations. The medical doctor did a good job of keeping me mentally off guard and mentally stupid. The surgeon had something else in mind for me on the actual day of surgery, a mental and cosmetic whammy.

How was I supposed to know that the medical doctor and cosmetic surgeon was setting me up for something diametrically opposite of what I wanted and needed cosmetically? I was hunting for the right surgeon, and this doctor was hunting me for his own selfish agenda. These facts have become more evident to me as the years have gone by.

The doctor who I was questioning before surgery didn't have the cosmetic skills or the discernment to rightly interpret my cosmetic interests. I was being mentally worked on by an eccentric predator.

A friend of mine in Lincoln, Arkansas, told me recently, "A shark doesn't negotiate. It just comes up and takes your leg off."

Postsurgery, the painful and devastating results became more and more evident with the passing of time. I wondered and questioned over and over in my mind how this could have happened to me. I felt like I had been violated by a medical surgeon who should have never touched my nose and ears.

The doctor's approach even caught me off guard on the very day of surgery. Postsurgery, my mind was black and dismally blank with the powerful effects of his cosmetic heist that had been forced on my mental faculties and facial features. The reader may conclude that I was stupid for going to a cosmetic surgeon who I came to realize sometime after surgery was not listed with any of the twenty-four boards of medical specialists, ABMS. I didn't realize what Dr. Cutter's qualifications were when I went in for an initial consultation. I had learned from a woman who works for a board-certified plastic surgeon in the Pacific Northwest and answered my phone call that, "Cosmetic surgery is an enhancement of a person's appearance. Plastic surgery focuses on repairing and reconstructing possibly abnormal structures." I didn't know these facts and other revealing things about Dr. Cutter before surgery. Maybe I was being unknowingly naive at the time, but I thought I was being an honest and active realist in my pursuit for the right surgeon who could do exactly and precisely what I desired cosmetically.

Postsurgery I have learned that Dr. Cutter can reconstruct the face under his dental license, DDS; and under his MD, medical license he can practice plastic surgery. According to the staff member who answered my call to the MQAC, Dr Cutter "has a general anesthesia permit under his dentistry." I also learned postsurgery that "a medical doctor does not have to be board certified in the state of Washington to practice medicine."

Postsurgery I gradually came to realize that I had been royally ripped off cosmetically and financially by a cosmetic predator.

Years before I went to see Dr. Cutter, who I found out postsurgery was a doctor of medicine, MD, and a doctor of dental surgery, DDS, as a dentist, I had a woman who worked for a prominent plastic surgeon in the Pacific Northwest inform me that when it came to plastic surgery, you want a double-board plastic surgeon. A board-certified plastic surgeon sent me an e-mail saying, "doubled-board means certified in two specialties: general surgery and plastic ophthalmology and plastic ent and plastic reconstruction surgery." Regretfully I had forgotten all about that good advice. Dr. Cutter was not the board-certified plastic surgeon who was listed with any of the twenty-four boards of medical specialties that I needed and was searching for. Unfortunately I also found out postsurgeries that Dr. Cutter was not the board-certified reconstructionist that I wanted for my specific facial feature needs. I learned postsurgeries that Dr. Cutter is double-board-certified, but he is not a specialist in the nose and ears, as the American Board of Medical Specialties' true surgeons are.

Years later, I again went on a quest for the right surgeon for me. The approach Dr. Cutter (not his real name) took with me was just like that of a smooth-talking salesman who did not want me to focus on what I was about to purchase. A slick car salesman doesn't want you to think about how you are going to make your payments, nor does he take the time to get to know you personally as an individual. If he is only interested in advancing his salesmanship status, he probably won't invest the time to find out your likes and dislikes in searching for the right car just for you. I assumed that if Dr. Cutter couldn't do what I wanted and needed for my cosmetic interests, he would be considerate enough to refer me to a more qualified surgeon, but my assumption was wrong because Dr. Cutter had his own cosmetic plans and vision for my facial features.

I had had previous surgeries for my nose, ears, and chin, so I was very particular about finding the right cosmetic surgeon for myself. Prior to having any surgeries, I had seen an ad in the yellow pages regarding how to find the right surgeon for your cosmetic needs. When I called the phone number, the young woman who answered told me that cosmetic surgeons and plastic surgeons are basically the same, and so I started on my quest for the right surgeon for me.

The reason for my book is that I care about people and I would like to save hopeful cosmetic consumers the mental anguish and the painful cosmetic devastation that I experienced back in the nineties.

During that decade I had my cosmetic dreams actually destroyed by a sociopath. He had told me only so much before the surgery, and he began to make up things subsequent to my multiple surgeries postsurgery. I realize now that I had met the wrong cosmetic surgeon, who never recognized my cosmetic wants or needs for my facial features. That is more than scary. It was a truly painfully devastating experience that began to plunge my life into a deep sea of bewildering questions, and it slowly began to destroy my self-esteem and self-image as a unique creation of God. Dr. Cutter was not the board-certified plastic surgeon that I was searching for, although he performed surgeries on my facial features in the nineties.

I watched a television program one day about plastic surgery. The narrator commented that every year there are ten thousand cases of cosmetic surgery that are unnecessary. I know for a 100 percent fact that my cosmetic fiasco was totally unnecessary, and I now realize that it was clearly a cosmetic and financial crime. I had concluded that my particular case was a cosmetic homicide, but for years I wasn't able to figure out what Dr. Cutter had done to plunder my cosmetic and financial business. I had repeatedly requested a new hearing with the Medical Quality Assurance Commission, the medical board that issued Dr. Cutter's medical license, MD, and the Dental Quality Assurance Commission, the dental board that issued his DDS license. The above commissions govern Dr. Cutter's licensing to remain in practice.

I had sent in a series of complaint letters to the dental licensing board, DQAC, and to the medical licensing board, MQAC, over a period of years requesting legal action to be taken against Dr. Cutter. I also requested a reconsideration for a new hearing against the medical doctor calling for his licensing to be revoked or for disciplinary action to be taken against him. I would be willing to post these requests on my website so that the readers may read for themselves of my plea for help through a new hearing, justice, and a criminal investigation and action to be taken against Dr. Cutter for his crimes committed against me. I became convinced beyond a shadow of a doubt that medical malpractice and criminal actions by Dr. Cutter had truly been committed against me, and I wanted the iron will of justice to prevail against him. I assumed that after my complaints Dr.

Cutter would be held liable for his cosmetic and financial crimes against me. I was absolutely wrong in my assumption.

I found out sometime later postsurgery when I happened to inquire of the Medical Quality Assurance Commission that Dr. Cutter wasn't even requested to respond to my complaint letters nor to the commission's inquiries concerning the approach that he had taken toward me. This medical doctor utilized piracy of my cosmetic hopes and financial business, and he wasn't required to explain his abnormal psychology to the review boards. Each year that I requested an investigation regarding my cosmetic case, it ended up with a denial of my request. I didn't experience a reputable plastic surgeon working on my facial features, but medical negligence, malpractice, and utter butchery by the wrong cosmetic surgeon.

I was robbed big-time.

Before anyone ever begins his or her search for the right cosmetic or plastic surgeon for himself or herself, they will want to read *The Ultimate Violation*. I, Kurtess Scone, am living testimony against a malicious cosmetic predator who had disguised himself as a caring medical surgeon.

THE DOUBLE MIRROR

I, Kurtess Lief Scone, grew up in Lupine, a small town in a region of the Pacific Northwest, with my family of six, consisting of one brother, two sisters, and my mother and father. My Christian parents' pastorate was a small work among the American Indian congregation at the Lupine Assembly of God Church. The Lord had blessed the Scone family ministry among the small congregation throughout the years.

My father, Benjamin, and my mother, Jessica, had me and my siblings dedicated to the Lord as babies for God's use and service. Jessica remembers how I as a young boy fell off the front-row pew being fast asleep and how I continued right on sleeping on the floor as the church service kept on moving. I showed a remarkable comfortableness in the house of prayer, and I never cried out whenever I would fall onto the floor.

Jessica learned from the doctor that I was born with a children's disease named rickets. In this disease, because of a lack of vitamin D or sunlight, the bones often are characterized by being soft or even bent. Jessica began giving me a bone-strengthening product called Bone Meal, which the doctor had recommended to help strengthen my weak bones by giving me the necessary chemical element of vitamin D that my young body needed to grow a strong skeletal structure. I had difficulties trying to walk as well as a child my age, and naturally my mother was concerned about the weakness caused by the childhood ailment I physically inherited. I found that it was difficult to walk until I was approximately three years of age. With the Lord's overseeing protection and the doctor's advice to use vitamin D supplements, I continued to grow into a healthy young boy.

I had a severe ear infection as a young child, and my mother prayed for me to be healed. The Lord Our Healer, Jehovah Rapha, reached down His gracious hand of compassion and healed me of my ear infection at a tender age. I have continued to have excellent hearing throughout the years, and I have not had a serious ear infection of this type since. My caring father and mother made sure that all of their children were prayed for, regardless of what ailed them at the time. As loving parents, they positively wanted their children to continue to have God's strong protection and divine health for their future well-being as well.

One day, the family stopped to see the nearby rapid-flowing Celway River and its large boulders. The rushing river was capped with white water, and as the Scone family was viewing the spectacular scenery, I went back to the car and crawled onto the backseat to go to sleep. When the family members couldn't find me anywhere, they became extremely concerned that I might have fallen into the powerfully rushing watercourse. To their surprise, they returned to the car to find me resting comfortably on the backseat without a concern for the greatness of the wonders of nature. After all, to me, getting some necessary sleep was a more important matter at the time than the family's interest in the great outdoors.

I discovered as a young boy that I took an interest in God's creation as a visible witness to nature's wonders. God's handiwork is clearly evident by the things that He has created, and I fully enjoyed the creatures that He had created. The Holy Bible tells us that we are fearfully and wonderfully made as God's marvelous creation.

When I was five years old, the Scone family moved to Clover Valley, the city where I was born. One warm summer day, as I was catching butterflies in a vacant field about five blocks from my home, a big bully stole the butterflies from me. It didn't matter to the larger boy that I had worked ever so patiently at catching the butterflies and had carefully placed them into a paper-cup bucket. The big kid decided what had belonged to me was now his to take. I was hurt by this act of aggression on the part of the adversary; however, feeling inferior due to my size, I didn't offer any resistance. I hadn't learned to fight for what rightfully belonged to me.

When I first moved to Clover Valley, I slept downstairs in the basement along with my brother, Daniel. One night, I found that I needed to go to the bathroom. Still new to the home, I made the trek up the basement stairs, turned to the right, and opened the door, ready to take aim to fire in the hole.

Unfortunately, the hole was in our living room coat closet. My mother, Jessica, caught me just in the nick of time and quickly took me down the hallway to the bathroom on the right. I wasn't aiming to displease when I took aim at the wrong dark hole. I was still foggy from sleep, and I needed a motherly hand to lead me down the hallway to the right watering hole or thunder mug. I never had another problem with finding the bathroom from that day on.

One day I decided to catch honeybees that were buzzing around a honeysuckle bush next to my family home. I was successfully catching the honeybees and placing them into a glass jar until I got stung on my arm by one of the insects. I removed the stinger and was willing to have another go at catching honeybees for a while longer. My mother asked me what I was going to do with the honeybees. I told her that the bees were going to make honey for me and that I was going to make some money.

As a young boy, I never did make any money at catching honeybees for a living, but I know that certain people are successful at making money raising honeybees in beehives. I have enjoyed having a peanut butter and honey sandwich now and then throughout the years. I recognize that pure honey goes well with a lot of things.

During my boyhood, I enjoyed having pets in my home. My mother bought me a turtle that I liked to play with after school. I also enjoyed having a multicolored parakeet that the family named Pretty Pete. I looked forward to coming home after school and spending time trying to teach my parakeet to talk. I would talk to him in his cage, and also in the restroom in front of the bathroom mirror.

I was able to teach Pretty Pete to say, "Pretty bird." Pretty Pete grew accustomed to riding around on my shoulder inside our home. When I worked on my homework after school, Pretty Pete would come flying down and land on my pencil as I worked on my assignments. Pretty Pete liked to land on the family table or land into my bowl, and I would keep right on eating my cereal.

I grew accustomed to spending time with Pretty Pete, and I also became acquainted with sensing my parakeet's feet on top of my hair. One day Pretty Pete died from the flu, and I and my best friend, Treat Munson, gave the bird a decent burial behind our family home. Treat and I placed Pretty Pete into a plastic butter container and lowered him down into his grave. After covering dirt over his plastic casket, we gave Pretty Pete a three-gun salute with my Downing Rifle BB gun. Treat then placed a cross at Pretty Pete's grave site, symbolizing his Christian burial.

As a young boy, I discovered that I enjoyed the female gender of the human species; God had created them so they could become wonderful friends with young boys. I especially liked a tall girl in my first grade named Connie. I decided to stop by the corner grocery store to buy some candy before going to Connie's house to see if she could come out to play with me. I spent twenty-five cents on candy at the store, which was a lot of money to spend on a girl back in the sixties. Your money was able to buy much more candy than you can today. I knocked at Connie's front door, and when I found out that she couldn't come out to play, I walked home eating all the candy in my sack by myself. My mother had thought that I might break a tooth biting down on the hard jawbreakers. Thank goodness I didn't break any of my teeth, but my mouth certainly got a good workout chewing all the candy by myself. Although I liked to play with Connie at school, I never was successful at becoming her steady boyfriend. When I grew up, I came to recognize that the Lord's will for our ongoing spiritual growth is to only date Christians.

I recall how I and my friends liked to shoot yellow jackets with our homemade rubber-band guns after the Sunday morning service. Our escapades with the bright yellow-marked hornets, found way high up, on, or around the upper beams of the Weeler Assembly of God Church in another region of the Pacific Northwest, were quite daring. It was risky business to shoot one of these potential multiple-stinging large insects, but the boys found the thrill to be well worth the risk. We were able to bring down a few of them whenever we persisted at shooting our rubber bands at these flying insects. Should the boys get tired of trying to bring down the yellow jackets, we could go outside to the back of the church and walk down to the East Fork of Silver Tip Grizzly Creek to try to catch crawdads, frogs, or garter snakes.

Another activity the young boys enjoyed doing together was walking over several blocks from the church to the train tracks, where we could throw rocks at the birds sitting on the power lines overhead. One day I was successful at hitting one of the birds with my quick throwing arm. There were positively fun things to do in between church services on Sundays for me and my friends.

One Sunday night after church, I discovered a nicely wrapped present inside the family's front screen door. When I saw who the gift was from, I decided to return the special favor by giving this real nice girl named Angela what I considered at the time an unusual present.

I placed a large bottle of Pepsi and some hard candy inside an empty shoe box and wrapped it up the best that I could. I took it up to Angela's house at night and left it on her front porch next to her front door.

After I got back home, I opened Angela's gift to me and found that she had given me a *Password* game. I became embarrassed as I reflected upon the difference in value that my gift would have cost and the value of Angela's gift to me. I decided to take a classmate friend with me and go to the store after school the next day to buy Angela a higher-priced gift to balance out the cost of our gifts to each other. My friend picked out a facial powder product and some perfume. As I left these additional gifts for Angela, I hoped that this would finalize our gift exchange. I didn't hear anything from Angela about whether she liked or didn't like my gift, so I concluded that I had effectively brought the gift giving to an end.

I had a dog named Elijah that I kept chained up outside of the house. On one occasion, my best friend, Treat, came over to show his new sweater to me, and Elijah jumped up and ripped a hole in Treat's new sweater with his front claws. Treat was so hurt by the dog's excited action that he decided to go home early for the day.

Another time the Scone family had a dog named Leakalou. The animal wet so many times as a puppy that Marlie, my sister, thought we should change the dog's name to Leakalake. The dog got distemper on Christmas Eve one year, and our father took it down to the dog pound, where they put the animal to sleep.

Later I had a wonderful solid black dog the family called Nubbin because of his short tail. I had heard that Nubbin was a terrier, but he looked like a shrunken Labrador retriever with a short tail. Nubbin grew up to be lively dog, with a big heart for me. When Nubbin was a puppy, I kept him in my bedroom at night. As Nubbin grew up, although he was still small in size, my mother wanted him to be chained up outdoors. Nubbin reluctantly went along with this plan, but he loved to play and be with me all the time. Nubbin was a great pet for me, and we enjoyed spending a lot of time together.

My friends and I liked to play hide-and-seek with Nubbin. We would throw a bone or a ball down the street, and then run and try to hide from Nubbin. Nubbin would run the object down and retrieve it in his mouth and then diligently track the boys down, whether we were hiding in a tree, behind a car, or up a telephone pole. Nubbin had excellent tracking skills and a keen sense of smell.

One day Treat and I threw the bone down the street and quickly hightailed it behind a neighbor's house without stopping. We continued to run through two neighbors' backyards and then across the street, only to make another fast run across another street and a dash up the alley for approximately one hundred feet. Treat and I then ran into a vacant lot and hid behind a storage shed. We sat down to rest from all of our running, thinking that we had outsmarted and successfully hid from Nubbin this time. A short time later, we observed Nubbin slowly running with his nose to the ground. When our trail ran cold, Nubbin turned around, and discovered Treat and I hiding out behind the shed.

One day the Scone family went to Sam's Lake to go boating and waterskiing. I was inexperienced at waterskiing. As I put out three separate large sprays of water, I lost my balance on the skis, sending me crashing into the lake. When Nubbin saw me fall into the lake, he entered the water and began swimming out to rescue the fallen skier. My mother called out to Nubbin to come back to shore, being concerned for his safety, and Treat, who was an excellent swimmer, started swimming out after Nubbin. Treat was successful in grabbing Nubbin by the tail and getting him turned around, guiding him back to the beach. Nubbin was a great swimmer, and had he been left to swim the distance out to where I was in the lake, he would have succeeded in doing so. I wasn't a good swimmer as a boy, so I ended up riding in the boat back to the shoreline where the others were looking on.

Nubbin was a great dog for retrieving a stick or a ball that I or one of my friends would throw out into a lake or into a slow-moving part of the Sussan or Big Rock Rivers. As I held onto my dog's short tail, Nubbin would pull me around on a lake or pond as I lay on an inner tube or an air mattress. Nubbin was always good about lending his availability, willingness, and helping tail.

Nubbin was my favorite pet and would do anything he physically could for me. One winter day at my request, my mother, Jessica, made a halter for Nubbin to wear. I was then able to hitch Nubbin to my sled to provide a ride for me. Nubbin wouldn't pull me on the sled until I walked him up to the next street and then told him to go home. When Nubbin heard the command to go home, he dug his paws into the snow, and with great effort, he began pulling me all the way home on my sled. I loved my special dog, Nubbin, that provided faithful companionship for me as a boy.

Just like Mary and her little lamb, wherever I went, Nubbin wished to go along with me. For Nubbin's own protection and for my personal privacy, I occasionally told my dog to stay home in a stern voice. Nubbin had been consistently trained to obey my commands to come or to stay home whenever I told him to do so.

Nubbin provided a lot of entertainment value with his relationship to my friends and me. One afternoon Nubbin was sprayed with pepper spray by the mailman. When he entered the Scone family home after being sprayed, he began rubbing his eyes with his paws to get rid of the stinging spray. Daniel and a friend of his with protruding ears came into the house, and when Nubbin observed Daniel's friend, he fell off the couch rubbing his eyes.

My friend Treat and I were home from school, and when we witnessed Nubbin fall off the couch rubbing his eyes after looking at Daniel's friend, we began to laugh at the situation. Thank goodness Daniel and his friend had gone downstairs; hopefully they weren't offended by our laughter. Eventually the pepper spray wore off, and Nubbin was back to being a good dog again and acting like himself once more.

Nubbin discovered that whatever I liked to eat was good enough for him to eat, too. I would give Nubbin a portion of bread with peanut butter spread on it. When Nubbin opened his mouth to take the bite of sandwich, I would clamp down on his muzzle with my hands. After lifting my hands from Nubbin's muzzle, I would stand back and watch my dog have a challenging chewing exercise. I could be a rascal to Nubbin; being such a good dog, Nubbin didn't deserve it. At times I would give Nubbin a Sugar Daddy sucker to chew and chew on. As a natural consequence, Nubbin acquired a sweet tooth. My friends and I would be amused at poor Nubbin's chewing ordeals. I discovered that Nubbin was an excellent fielder of French toast, pancakes, meat, or candies that I would toss his way.

Daniel was not fond of Nubbin watching him eat at the dinner table. He felt Nubbin keenly staring at his every bite of food until finally he couldn't take it anymore. He suddenly stopped eating and said to Nubbin, "Go on, vulture." Daniel wasn't compassionate toward Nubbin's steady hunger plight. I fed Nubbin's hungry stomach daily, but unless Nubbin was completely stuffed, he always seemed to be ready for more food. Nubbin was able to eat a lot more than you'd expect looking at his small size.

When Nubbin had been chained up outdoors at night, unknown to the Scone family, the paper carrier had teased him repeatedly. My mother, Jessica, finally caught the paper carrier dangling his paper bag in front of Nubbin just outside the reach of Nubbin's taut chain. Jessica stopped by the paperboy's home to have a talk with his mother and reported the mischievous actions of her son toward Nubbin. The paperboy had a sudden change of behavior when he delivered the paper from then on, but Nubbin's dislike for the paperboy never went away. Nubbin continued to growl and bark at him as if he could eat him alive for breakfast.

I discovered that Nubbin had a strong dislike for the mailman as well. Nubbin instinctively knew the time of day that the mailman would make his afternoon delivery to our home. One day the front door was open, and Nubbin managed to push the screen door open. He immediately went running down past the side lot and began barking and growling intensely at the mail carrier.

With Nubbin eagerly waiting just outside of the gate to the next-door neighbor's fence, the mailman saw his opportunity to settle the score with the angry dog. He decided to cure Nubbin of ever giving him a hard time again and put a stop to Nubbin's ever biting him on the leg in the future. With Nubbin angrily growling and barking with intensity in front of the gate, the mailman kicked as hard as he could into the wooden gate, which should have slammed into the face and body of the fierce canine. But to his painful surprise, the neighbor's gate didn't move one inch under the powerful impact of the mailman's foot.

The mailman had momentarily forgotten that it was the kind of gate that needs to be opened by pulling it inward, not pushing it outward. If only the gate had cooperated with the mailman's actions, Nubbin could have ended up seriously hurt. My father, Benjamin, talked to the mailman about trying to make friends with the dog. The mailman said that he didn't have time to make friends with dogs.

My boyhood dog Nubbin could be considered a wonder dog by today's standards. Nubbin was not only my special dog; he was the best dog that I ever owned. Nubbin was a dedicated, affectionate, vigorous companion and friend to me, and he was always eager to go along with whatever I wanted to do or wherever I wanted to go. Nubbin was considered a part of the Scone family. One summer the Scone family traveled to North Dakota to visit the old family homestead and our relatives, who lived on a wheat farm. Nubbin had to be given sleeping pills to subdue his nervousness for him to safely travel in comfort.

To protect the car seats from Nubbin's claws, he was given rubber boots to wear. When Nubbin was let out of the car to do his business, he looked awkward walking or running with the rubber boots on. He seemed very uncomfortable and awkward wearing his rubber boots, like Pluto, the cartoon character in Walt Disney animated films. He definitely would have shaken them right off his paws if he could have. Nubbin managed to survive the trip to see our relatives, though, and also to see Yellowstone National Park.

It was pretty neat to have a bear cub leave its paw print on the '69 four-door Chevrolet car window as a souvenir for my family to show friends when we returned home. The Scone family vacation was a good one for both Nubbin and me to go on together.

My friends and I liked to look for fun and exciting things to do. Treat and I liked to watch *The Outside Sportsman Show,* with Kurt Gowdy as the narrator. After watching an exciting edition about big-game hunting on the sportsman show, Treat and I wanted to go hunting for the Scone family's pet cat, named Bo. The Scones had a good black-and-white cat that became our unwilling big-game mountain lion. I would tell Nubbin to find the cat, and Nubbin eagerly knew what I wanted him to do.

Nubbin, Treat, and I would take off hunting down Bo as if we were tracking down a big-game mountain lion right in the mountains of the Scone family yard, side lot, or neighbor's yard somewhere. Nubbin would act out his natural tracking abilities and diligently lead myself and Treat right to the exact hiding place of Bo. Upon seeing Nubbin, Bo would be off and running for his life. Nubbin would be in hot pursuit of the family pet and do a great job of getting the cat treed, just like hound dogs treeing a mountain lion into a holding position up a tree or boxed into a cave. The big-game hunting experiences were exciting for the boys after watching each sportsman program, but it was an unpleasant experience for Bo, the family's peaceful feline, every time.

I recall one night when Nubbin had a sad encounter with a black-and-white creature down the street from the Scone family home. While the family was outside of the house talking together, Nubbin went after an animal in the dark of night. To him it may have looked like a cooperative cat to chase after, but he discovered that this black-and-white animal sprayed him with a liquid perfume that left him smelling foul, a horrible stinking smell. When Nubbin came back home after his personal encounter with the skunk, my mother, Jessica, wanted me to give my dog a good bath to rid my pet of the horrible-smelling stench. Jessica had canned fruit for years, and she wanted me to open a couple of jars of tomatoes stored on the basement shelf to get rid of the stink. I was not happy with Nubbin's choice of dark encounters with an animal that might look like a black-and-white cat, but positively doesn't turn and run when an intense dog that doesn't have the good sense to leave it alone chases after it in the heat of the night.

I was going into the sixth grade the next day, and I didn't want to go to school smelling like a skunk. I was concerned about the horrific stench getting onto my clothes when I brought Nubbin into the house. However, I took Nubbin into the bathroom and turned on the bathwater, subsequently pouring a couple of large jars of tomatoes into the bathtub. I did my best to scrub Nubbin down with the acidic juices contained in the canned tomatoes. I hoped my dog had learned his lesson after the pathetic encounter with the backside of a creature looking similar to Bo, the Scone family pet cat. Only this creature had a white stripe down its back, and not all over its body mixed with black patches, as Bo had.

One day, I was helping to paint my grandparents' home, which my mother had inherited upon her parents passing away. Nubbin and I were on our way back home on foot. I had already crossed over a busy thoroughfare in Clover Valley, and I was quickly heading for home. When I didn't find Nubbin right by my side or following safely behind, I turned around to look for him. I saw Nubbin hit by a truck on the busy road of Cloverland Street, which suddenly became Grief Street for me. I couldn't believe this had happened to my most loyal friend. I reached down and picked up my lifeless best friend and pet, and sadly carried his body home with me. I cried deeply over the death of my favorite pet and requested that the Lord raise him up from the dead so that I could continue to have a loving relationship with my dog.

The Lord never answered my prayer to give life back to my dog, but He would continue to be good and faithful to me in other ways. I didn't want another dog to take Nubbin's place because I knew that there wouldn't ever be a more special pet that provided such faithful, good, and loyal companionship to me as Nubbin.

I had a self-confidence derived from my multitalented family. My father, Benjamin, was a good pastor, a barber, and an excellent musician.

My older brother, Daniel, was a multitalented athlete who had worked with me as his younger brother to improve myself as an individual athlete. Our mother had said to Daniel, "You can do whatever you put your mind to." Daniel was good in baseball and basketball as a junior high athlete. Daniel ran in track when he was in high school only as a means to pursue his love for the sport of basketball at Clover Valley High School. In his senior year, Daniel was voted captain of the track team, and he was voted most inspirational of the varsity basketball team.

Carol became a good piano player as a youth, and she was an excellent student throughout her years in school. Marlie grew up to become an excellent piano player who played by ear. She was also a good singer and good actor when entertaining people. Marlie was especially recognized for her acting role as Ernestine at the Tabernacle Church in Graniteville. I appreciated hearing Carol, Marlie, and Benjamin sing and play gospel songs together. On different occasions Benjamin and Jessica would either sing a duet or sing independently at Christian churches we would travel to when my parents were given an invitation to come and share in gospel and song with the congregation.

I received significance in life as an individual created in the image of God. God gave me abilities and talents that I have used for God's glory. My confidence received a real boost in life when my talent of being a good baseball pitcher was consistently validated by my coach, players, and family members.

I fondly remember the Scone family playing music together and how our family's talents were used to bring honor to God in Christian churches. I came to realize that I had many good qualities in life going for me in my personal life. I recognized that how we see ourselves is a reflection of how we look at others. I had faith in God, had good qualities, and had good friends to do things with.

My family would hold hands and start the day by saying a prayer together. I remember one of the family prayers that we would say at the dinner table:

> *Come, Lord Jesus, be our guest. May this food by thee be blessed. Amen.*

I was not totally familiar with the family prayer as a boy, and I would pray it this way:

> *Come, Lord Jesus, be our guest. May this day by BB blest. Amen.*

Marlie said to me that I was purposely getting the words wrong, but since I was young, I honestly didn't know the right wording of the prayer. Kids can easily misjudge one another. They may not properly understand their brother or sister, who may not know what they think the sibling should know. It's easy to believe that we are always right as seen through our own rose-colored glasses, and that's why kids say what they say to each other. There are a lot of times, as children and later as adults, that we have our own preconceived notions and ideas about people and our personal relationships with others.

As a boy, I, in retrospect, needed to have more knowledge, better understanding regarding life and relationships, and greater wisdom concerning how to deal with my personal relationships with my family and friends. I continued to grow and increase in maturity and wisdom before God and man with the passing of the years.

I had character developed in my life as a young boy growing up in a Christian home. Whenever I heard one of my non-Christian friends take God's name in vain by using His name as a swear word, it would bother me. I was known by my friends as someone who didn't swear. I was pretty well accepted by my family and the good Christian churches that I attended while growing up, which placed a high premium on and respect for Biblical teachings that were to be observed according to the laws of God.

It was understood in the Scone family that God's Word was extremely important, and that His commands, laws, and principles were not to be broken or violated. Unfortunately we are seeing today the tragedies of people's broken lives because they erroneously believe that they can sin by breaking God's laws with impunity without experiencing serious consequences in their personal lives and in their bodies.

Some powerful examples of law-breaking consequences can be clearly seen in the teenage pregnancies, AIDS, alcohol, and drug abuse crises in the United States of America.

As the Holy Bible says, "A man shall reap whatever he sows. . . . And be sure your sin will find you out" (Gal. 6:7; Num. 32:23). There are God's laws, man's laws, and nature's laws set in this present world, and we need to respect each and every one of them for our own good.

I remember one Sunday when the small congregation were seeking God at the altar and in the front pews at the Weeler Assembly of God Church, where my parents ministered in another valley. Pastor Benjamin Scone had concluded his sermon, in which he urged the congregation to seek the Lord Jesus for the powerful experience of the baptism of the blessed Holy Spirit. I remember seeking the Lord the best way that I knew of, by the example of others who were seeking the Lord at the same time.

Everyone was kneeling in prayer at the altar or on the steps leading to the platform of the church. Each one was calling upon the name of the Lord God in earnest heartfelt prayer. I remember crying at the altar at the tender age of eleven; at the time, I felt that it was an emotionally sensitive and spiritual experience for myself.

I discovered that once I got back home, I could tell dirty stories to my friends just as bad as the best of them. I had not experienced the big change from my time of seeking God at the altar with the other Christians at the Weeler Assembly of God Church that the Lord would provide for me one day during my adolescent years.

I am grateful that my father didn't pursue having a barbershop in Weeler, located in the Pacific Northwest, to generate more income along with his pastorate when he was considering moving the Scone family to live in Weeler. I never heard that my siblings were in favor of moving from Clover Valley to Weeler, where our parents had talked about moving the family. The family as a whole would not have approved of the move to a small logging community over living in Clover Valley.

One day Treat Munson and I were throwing rocks at an old, black, cast-iron stove in the lot of the St. Paul's Catholic School building. I bent down to pick up some more rocks to throw and happened to lift my head up in the line of fire as Treat hurled another rock at the old cooking utensil. I took a hard hit to the back of my head as the rock slammed into me squarely in the center of the back of my head.

As I walked home several blocks away, I kept my head down because I was bleeding from a head wound. My mother, Jessica, asked me to let her know if I began seeing double. Thank goodness for me, I didn't see double after the rock-throwing episode, but I recognized that I hadn't used my head when it came to throwing rocks that day. I realized that not using my head to think correctly about what my friend was doing at the time is not how one gets ahead in life.

I was enjoying a new bow and arrows that my mother had purchased for me when I decided to take aim at what I thought was a rat in back of Treat's home. The creature was in a dried sticky bush just behind the backyard fence. I could see that the little animal had stopped moving in the bush. I let go of my arrow, and wham, it struck the four-footed creature in its side, piercing it deeply.

The animal began making a crying, screeching sound of pain. I discovered to my horror that what I had thought was a rat that most cats would catch turned out to be a small, baby bunny rabbit. I felt bad about shooting the bunny rabbit, and I then wished I could catch the soft, furry, long-eared animal to take home as a pet.

After I removed the arrow, hoping the rabbit would recover from its wound, the little animal didn't live long. The bunny rabbit was the only animal that I killed with my bow and arrow during my life. I regretted killing the light brown bunny rabbit in the act of a mistaken identification of a different creature, which has been recognized as a health hazard with deadly consequences in American history.

I recall taking my friend Treat to a Christian evangelistic meeting, where David Wilkerson was preaching the gospel of Christ Jesus. I was not gloriously saved myself, being just a boy when I heard the good news about Jesus Christ, the Savior of mankind. After David Wilkerson, the mighty man of God, had preached a powerful sermon about the good news of God's wonderful salvation, he invited anyone who would like to receive Jesus Christ into their heart and life to come forward during the altar call to accept the Lord. I remember how my good friend Treat mentioned that he wanted to go forward, but he wanted me to go up front with him. I didn't feel like going forward even though I probably should have gone.

When I look back on that important moment in time, I positively recognize that I should have responded to the invitation, especially for my friend's sake. Treat did not go forward that day when the evangelist David Wilkerson gave the salvation invitation. The last time that I shared with my friend concerning the things of Christ Jesus years later, I found that Treat's heart was cold and indifferent to the things of the Lord.

I regret not going forward with my friend Treat for God's free gift of salvation when the Lord Jesus was knocking at his heart's door. If only we could roll back time, things could have been different for Treat and me on that golden day of opportunity.

Jesus says, "Behold, I stand at the door and knock. If anyone hears my voice and opens the door, I will come in to him and dine with him, and he with me" (Rev. 3:20). "For He says: 'In an acceptable time I have heard you, And in the day of salvation I have helped you.' Behold, now is the acceptable time, behold, now is the day of salvation" (2 Cor. 6:2).

At the time of David Wilkerson's Christian evangelistic crusade, I wasn't aware of these two powerful Bible verses that could have made a difference in my best friend, Treat Munson, possibly receiving the gift of salvation when the opportunity of eternal choices was given by the evangelist for Christ.

May we never let an opportunity of priceless worth leave us empty of eternal values.

I would like the reader to keep in mind that in the face of eternity, when all is said and done during the course of a person's life, that only what's done for Christ Jesus will last for time and eternity.

"That can only be done through our faith in the finished work of Jesus Christ on the cross of Calvary. Not only for our salvation, but also for daily life long sanctification. This is the only place that the Holy Spirit can operate in" (Rom. 6:3-14, 8:1-2,11; Eph. 2:13-18; Gal. 6:14; 1 Cor. 1:17-18,21,23; 1Cor. 2:2; Col. 2:14-15; and Jude:1-3).

I was visiting on the phone one day with a friend, Bud, who gave me the above quote. He provided scripture to support his quote at a later date.

———

Treat and I decided to experiment with smoking tobacco. Treat's father, George, smoked a pipe at his home, and Treat liked the smell of the cherry-flavored pipe smoke. His mother, Sally, smoked Marlboro cigarettes, and Treat brought one or two of them over for us to experiment with. Treat didn't want to bring more cigarettes over to my home so that his mother wouldn't notice any of them missing.

Watching how Treat smoked his cigarette by inhaling, I didn't like the thought of inhaling the smoke into my lungs, partly because I didn't think it was the right thing to do and I didn't want to become addicted to the bad habit of smoking cigarettes. I became a willing participant of experimenting with tobacco smoking, though, as monkey see, monkey do. It was not a wise thing for a young Christian boy to be doing, and it was also not a smart thing for a good healthy athlete to be doing. Thank goodness I learned my lesson at an early age that cigarette smoking can be hazardous to a person's health.

My father, Benjamin, grew corn in a family garden in our side lot. Since my mother had a tobacco can on our back porch that had belonged to her father, Robert, we decided to use some of the tobacco from the can in our homemade corncob pipes.

Treat took time to bore out the middle of a corncob and make a hole in the base of the cob to provide room for the pipe mouthpiece. At first, we took turns smoking from the homemade pipe.

After we finished smoking the tobacco gently packed in the corncob pipe, I decided to fill the pipe again for a second round of smoking. When I began to smoke from the cob pipe the second time, I began to feel nauseous. I went down the alley and threw up; that sickening feeling had caused me to feel uncomfortable as a negative consequence of smoking tobacco. My body was telling me that smoking was not good for me.

Unfortunately for me, I tried out smoking cigars before I gave up the nasty smoking experimentation during my adolescent years. I am grateful to God that my smoking experimentation days didn't become a lifelong habit.

Life is a reflection of how we see ourselves, and it is true to life that how we see ourselves or the way we perceive ourselves can have a reflection in how we look at others. I found that I had high self-esteem and self-acceptance, and was willing to accept responsibility for my actions when I made mistakes.

I remember a time when a music teacher came to my first grade class. I sang out with great confidence, which caught the attention of the music teacher's ear.

When I performed well, singing with confidence or playing baseball well, at a young age, if rewarded by others I found that I wanted to continue the activity.

I learned the importance of having a competitive spirit in sports. As I look back on my childhood days, I can see that since my older brother put everything forth with the intention of executing high excellence, I wanted to imitate and model myself after what he had taught and demonstrated for me to do. When playing baseball, I endeavored to do my very best, and it left me with satisfying consequences as a result of my pitching performance on the mound. I later discovered that when I applied myself toward my music, my studies, or playing sports, I would naturally reflect the talents, gifts, and abilities that God had given to me. I have come to discover that my talents and abilities could positively help other people.

When I was a young boy, I thought that I was good looking in my own reflection of myself in the mirror. I felt that the opposite sex found me to be physically attractive as well.

I remember spending time in front of the mirror making different expressions with my mouth and nose trying to find the right look for me to make myself appear attractive for the girls at Cloverdale Elementary School.

My older sister, Carol, and her friends thought that I was a cute boy when I was young. I was a sensitive child growing up, and I remember that one of the girls that my brother liked didn't think that I was good looking as a boy.

Whenever I would hear a negative comment about my physical appearance from the opposite sex, it would make me feel rejected and deeply unattractive. I also felt self-conscious if a male friend or even someone I didn't know personally ever made a critical remark about my looks. One football coach made a cutting remark that I looked like a monkey. I took mental note of the coach's negative comment, but I kept on practicing on the football field along with the other players.

Any hurtful comment about my appearance caused me to become more self-conscious about my looks, but God helped me to have a healthy acceptance of myself. I could act shy around others that I didn't feel accepted by, but I would be nice toward other people that I didn't find physically attractive myself. I was willing to be sensitive toward the unlovely, as Jesus had done when He walked the earth.

I came to see myself as someone who was important to other people. My step-grandmother, Elma Jane Hillers, did her level best to make me believe that I was special. She would show her kind feelings toward me by baking a cherry pie for me. Elma Jane was greatly fond of me, and she always wanted to give me a slice of my favorite kind of pie each time I visited my grandparents.

I had an affectionate relationship with my mother, Jessica, and I liked to pat her pod (the belly fat on her stomach) when she would take time to make me eggs just the way I liked them or make me French toast on the kitchen stove. I especially appreciated my mother when she would make my favorite dessert, a whipped cream salad. My mother would ask me to slice the bananas or dates or grapes, and have me stir the whipping cream. I liked to express my physical affection for my mother for all the good and kindhearted things that she would do for me. I had my own reward system, and I knew exactly how to show my love and affection for the family members who made me feel good about myself. When I would pat my mother's pod as a skinny boy growing up in Clover Valley, Jessica would say, "Leave my fat alone. You just wait. One day you're going to be fat." I enjoyed showing affection to my mother, and Jessica appreciated receiving the fond attention from me as the youngest child.

I played fast-pitch baseball and fast-pitch softball. I was a very good pitcher on the teams that I played for. Each step of success gave me confidence at succeeding and achieving in competitive sports. My successes rewarded me with a feeling of satisfaction as an individual player and as a team player who was seen as a positive contribution to the team. Whenever I would lose a game for my team, I would take it personally pretty hard, and this would cause me to reflect heavily upon my own pitching performance and what I might have done wrong that may have contributed to my team's loss. I would always endeavor to pick myself up after a significant loss in order to make a positive difference in the next game.

One of the good players on the Little Aces baseball team was Tommy Ray, who played second base. Tommy was a good infielder at preventing any balls getting past him at his second-base position, and he was really good as a hitter as well. I remember going over to Tommy's place to see the rabbits they had outside in a large cage. They had several floppy-eared rabbits that I hadn't seen before. Tommy went to a school named St. Paul's Catholic School in Clover Valley. Tommy's and my friendship centered mostly around baseball, which included playing catch together or catching a ride to a game or practice with Jessica.

I recall one day when Tommy went inside of his house while I stayed outside by the rabbit cage. I discovered years later that my friend Tommy had gotten in trouble with the law for vandalizing cars and he was sent up to a juvenile detention center for boys. I also discovered years later that Tommy had been abused, along with his sisters, in their home by an alcoholic stepfather. I recall Tommy saying to me regarding the abuse in his home, "You never knew, Kurtess, did you?"

I responded to Tommy, "No, I never did."

I would become single-minded toward the things that I was interested in. I found that I put a great deal of focus and concentration onto playing baseball. I liked to watch the Oakland Athletics, the Boston Red Sox, and the Cincinnati Reds baseball teams on television because I liked watching good-quality pitching by some of the best major league pitchers.

I also enjoyed watching some of the best hitters going up against excellent pitching. I liked to watch Johnny Bench catch and throw out base runners with his quick releases to first, second, and third base. I would closely watch the pitching performances of these excellent pitchers so that I could learn to emulate their pitching examples, because I wanted to be successful at pitching at every level.

One summer day while I was with a friend at the Clover Valley baseball field, I discovered that there had been talk that I might be one of the best pitchers that ever came out of the local valley.

Whenever a young pitcher shows any signs of promise, some adults and young people begin talking about the possibility of him becoming a future sensation in the major leagues. With each young prospect who has any future hopes at succeeding in a particular sport, the general rule for intelligent adults and for the potential future prospect is that they must not get caught up in the emotional hype of the crowd of all ages.

There are a lot of variables that are susceptible to change, so everyone has to expect the best, wait and see, and follow each athlete's success and progress to hopefully emerge one day as a major league ball player. I would have enjoyed playing professionally as a major league pitcher if things had worked out in that direction.

I had a trusting nature about me regarding my relationship to other people. I grew up trusting that what my family said to me I could trust; I could expect them to keep their word. I had a simple, childlike faith and believed that I could depend on my family to honor their promises by keeping their commitments to me and to each other.

If my father, Benjamin, told our family that we needed to get to a church service on a certain day, the family members could expect him to take us to church that day.

If my mother, Jessica, agreed to take me to one of my baseball practices or to one of my games, I could trust that she would make certain that I would arrive at the ball field on time. I never learned in the Scone family not to trust individuals who had questionable or negative character qualities except for a couple of isolated cases that we knew of. One case dealt with the husband of a friend of my mother, who wanted my Christian parents to listen to demon spirits recorded on a record album. My mom told the man to take that record home or she would break it. I understand he was eventually admitted to a mental institution, as related to me later by my mother.

Distrust wasn't something that I learned a lot about in life because the local valley, and the surrounding area that I grew up in, was still largely a safe place to live.

I continued to trust in the good will of mankind for the common good of their fellow man. The Bible warns us to watch out for wolves in sheep's clothing, but I continued to have an innocent faith of trusting good people in positions of care and trust. I would one day have my innocent trust shattered by a person in a trusted position.

I recall one night when my sister Marlie and I went for a ride with our mother, Jessica, to get some skim milk for the family. Marlie and I discovered that the backseat could be pulled back so that we could crawl behind the backseat right into the trunk of our family car, a '48 Chevrolet. As we rode along in the trunk of the car, our mother didn't know what had happened to us until we came out from our hiding place.

I remember how I would go down with my father to the Arthers to pick up a gallon of milk, and how my dog Nubbin, when he was still alive, would run along on the sidewalk trying his level best to keep up with the slow-moving vehicle. We could hear Nubbin's claws clicking repeatedly on the pavement and concrete sidewalks. Since Nubbin was chained up outdoors on the north side of the Scone family home, I knew that Nubbin needed to get some exercise in order to stay healthy and physically fit. Years later, our family was blessed by being able to afford a new, modern, '59 automobile that Nubbin found was a good-running, slow-moving vehicle to run alongside. Nubbin was a great dog to take loping alongside when the family drove down to the Arthers for milk with our '59 Chevrolet.

I remember a time that I wanted to show my big sister Carol my blue-tailed lizard that I had gotten from a sandy field area on the north side of Clover Valley. I was pleased to be the proud owner of a blue-tailed lizard since they are extremely rare to come by.

Carol was intently reading an encyclopedia in the family's cushioned chair when I asked her if she would like to see my lizard. Carol didn't pay me any attention; it was as if she hadn't even heard a word I said to her. I eagerly inquired again if she would like to see my lizard.

Carol once more ignored my inquiry. Seeing that Carol wasn't listening to me, I was so anxious to show my big sister my blue-tailed lizard that I intentionally dropped the reptile directly on top of Carol's encyclopedia.

Carol became hysterical with fright and began screaming at the sight of the reptile. She literally started climbing up on top of the chair to get away from the lizard.

My oldest sister wanted me to get the lizard away from her, and I just wanted her to take a look at it. I couldn't believe how my sister Carol would have such a big fit over the likes of a tiny little creature. When I was questioned why I had frightened my sister like that, I said, "Man, I just wanted to show her my blue-tailed lizard."

I remember my sister Carol getting married when I was eleven years old to a man named Randell Wikum. Randell was a strong, tall man with blond wavy hair. She had met him at a Pentecostal Bible Institute in Browerland.

I was heartbroken that Carol wasn't going to marry Daniel's friend Randy, whom Carol had dated before she left for college. I cried about Carol's decision to marry a man I didn't know very well, and someone other than a personal friend of Daniel, who had become a friend to the Scone family household.

Carol made her decision to marry Randell because he fit the tall blond-haired man she had seen in her dreams. Carol had told Marlie one day, "I'm marrying a real man. He's nothing like our mealymouthed father." Carol didn't have the healthy respect toward our dad in her heart with love and honor that she ought to have had before she married Randell.

I had to get dressed up for the wedding, and then there were the family pictures that followed the wedding ceremony with the bride and groom. I recall that after the wedding, I enjoyed having punch, peanuts, and some of the wedding cake. I found that weddings can be nice to go to provided you get to enjoy the celebration with some tasty, good food and drinks at the reception.

I came to know Randell as an intelligent and friendly Christian man who thought pretty highly of himself, someone who was gifted with many talents that God had blessed him with. I would learn a lot more about Randell, a multitalented Christian man, in the future that I didn't know when I was growing up.

I recall how my friend Ernest liked for me to show my physical strength by giving Ernest piggyback rides. If I didn't show any interest in providing him a ride on my back, Ernest would entice me by offering to give me money for my back-carrying services.

Ernest liked to see what he could talk me into whenever I was with him, and one day he offered to give me a dollar if I would climb up the large locust tree situated in the yard on the south side of the Scone family house. I decided to take Ernest up on his profitable offer, and I went inside of our house to put on my big green coat and gloves that could protect me from the sticky thorns on my way up the large, shady tree.

Ernest pointed to the top of the tree, which I had to reach in order to be rewarded one greenback with a picture of George Washington on the front. I got less than eight feet up the trunk of the tree when I came to the realization that my climbing adventure was definitely not worth it. I decided to give up the climb. Ernest had himself a good laugh regarding my determination to climb the big tree before I had a change of mind early after embarkation on the adventure.

One day Ernest and I took turns putting on my large green coat in order to provide protection from being hit when we shot at each other with my Downing Rifle BB gun from across the street. On the west side of the neighbor's house were several trees that Ernest and I could use to shield ourselves momentarily from the small bronze-colored BBs being fired at one another as we kept moving along from tree to tree.

I remember how I took aim while timing it perfectly, and I hit Ernest with pinpoint accuracy right on my green coat. Ernest let out a sudden cry of pain, taking a direct hit from the hurtling BB. Ernest quickly came to the realization that he didn't want to get shot at anymore. After Ernest's turn with the BB gun, in which he was unsuccessful at hitting me with a BB, we came to a mutual agreement to stop the playing until another day.

I learned that my brother, Daniel, and his friends had gotten into a BB gunfight at the Viola Cemetery. It sounded like a real shoot-out had taken place as the older boys took turns firing BBs at one another from behind trees and various tombstones or any other nearby cover.

Ernest, and his brother Frank and I, along with our friend Joe, were shooting cows with BB guns down at the Willow's Packing Company. While we were intent on shooting at the cows inside the fences, some men from the packing company began running toward us. We took off over the fences to escape from being caught by the men only to find ourselves running right into being apprehended by the police, who were waiting for us beyond another fence. I, along with my friends, had our BB guns taken away from us by the Clover Valley police officers for our mischievous actions.

Randell Wikum, a police officer in Union, happened to be over visiting the Scone family when he witnessed my knees shaking as the police officer from Clover Valley was talking to my mother, Jessica, outside of our home about the cow-shooting incident.

I learned to have a healthy respect for the law during my adolescent years. I would eventually come to the realization that I needed the life-changing experience of the Lord Jesus Christ, who alone can make changes within the human heart and conscience of individuals.

I needed to get saved by faith in the grace of God extended through the precious blood of the Lord Jesus Christ to have the ongoing love and peace of God in my heart and life.

One night when I was a boy, Marlie, Daniel, and some of Daniel's friends wanted to play *Spotlight* outside the Scone family home. My oldest sister Carol happened to be inside the family home doing her homework while sitting on the couch.

We were having a good time playing outside when Marlie decided to go inside of the house to get a drink of water. Marlie was entering the home through the front door when she spotted a burglar with dark hair on the back porch. The intruder suddenly went out the back porch screen door and took off into the dark night air. Marlie told Daniel and his friends about the burglar, and they ran after the invader on foot as fast as they could run up the alleyway, searching diligently for the person who had entered our family home.

They were unsuccessful at finding the intruder that dark night, but that frightful incident put a scare into the Scone family. We knew that something more sinister could have happened to Carol if Marlie hadn't come in the home for a refreshing drink.

The Scone family believed that the good Lord protected Carol that night when she had been vulnerable to a potential assault by a burglar. This was the other case of evil intentions that the family was aware of.

"The angel of the Lord encamps all around those who fear Him, And delivers them" (Ps. 34:7 NKJV).

I was a friendly child, which made it easy for me to make friends in life. I found that when I would show myself friendly and take an interest in the interests and concerns of others, I found that I could make a friend of that person.

THE ULTIMATE VIOLATION

I enjoyed playing with Brian growing up; our families knew each other. I considered Treat Munson as my best friend among my boyhood friends whom I enjoyed spending time with.

Frank and Ernest White were brothers that I had spent a considerable amount of time with over the years, and one summer day I decided to join up with the White brothers on the east side of the Sussan River. My mother, Jessica, purchased me a blue pair of swimming fins. Frank and Ernest began teasing me about my new fins, and they told me that I couldn't catch them on their inner tubes. I took off chasing after them with my fins into the Sussan River. When I discovered that I was not going to be able to catch my friends, who were pulling away from me farther out into the river, I began to swim back toward the shore.

I was not considered the greatest swimmer in the world even with my new fins on. I remember stopping to secure one fin that was loose and how I looked at the shoreline that appeared so far away. I kept swimming toward the shore but stopped again to secure the other fin. I remember how tired I had become, and I began to wonder if I might drown by not making it back to shore. The next time that I stopped to rest, I discovered that I could touch the bottom, although I was still some distance from shore.

As I walked out of the river to rest on the shore, I found that my hands had cramped up on me, with my thumbs curling inward. My young life had been spared physical death, and I thank the good Lord for sparing my life.

I had taken swimming lessons when I was eight years old, but I didn't pass the test on the final lesson day at the Clover Valley swimming pool. I was going to be tested on swimming the width of the deep end, dog paddling without reaching up to touch or grab hold of the edge of the pool. Unfortunately, I failed the swimming class because I reached up and grabbed hold of the edge of the pool before I successfully reached the other side. I was disappointed with myself for failing the test, but I recognized that swimming was not my forte in life.

I enjoyed playing in the pool anyway. One day I was having a difficult time gasping for air inside of the swimming pool. I was close to the edge standing up, but the water was a little too deep for me and I wasn't able to pull myself up and out of the dangerous situation that I was in.

Thank goodness the lifeguard realized the predicament that I was in and reached down to rescue me from potentially drowning. God had used the lifeguard at the Clover Valley swimming pool to save my life that day.

I thank the good Lord for His protective hand on my life and for His guardian angels watching over me.

There was another time when I potentially could have drowned in a swift-flowing section of the Grand River. I had traveled up the Sussan River in a car with my friends to a section of the Grand River where the current was flowing at a faster pace. I walked out from the shoreline into a shallow but swift-flowing section of the river, and I didn't perceive the real danger until I tried to get back to shore. When I tried to swim back toward the shore, I found that the current was pulling me back out again. This time I gave it all I could muster and quickly swam toward the shore again. Thank God I was successful at reaching the shore, where I could stand up and walk onto the rock and sand area.

Once again, I found that my hands had cramped up, but I had escaped drowning. God had spared my life again. My parents, Benjamin and Jessica, had dedicated me to the Lord, as they had with all of their children, and I knew that God is the Divine Protector of each one of His children. I have come to realize that God wants to be our Savior, Rescuer, and Shock Absorber of the hurtful things in life. God is the giver of all good things that we have and everything that we enjoy in this life. When we come to recognize these wonderful truths, we can rest assured that He will watch over His children concerning our best interests in life.

My Adolescent Years

I grew up in a good Christian home in Clover Valley, in the Pacific Northwest. Life was not always easy for me during my adolescent years, but I can remember many good life-impacting experiences that happened in my Christian-based home that helped to develop the foundation of my character. I would experience many changes throughout my life that were positively constructive in building healthy, life-changing principles that would influence the direction of my life.

Although I had a good childhood, I was self-conscious about my appearance even at an early age. One day my big sister Marlie said to me, "Kurtess, you have a great big nose and a little bitty chin with little beady eyes." The words, spoken out of the blue, pierced me deeply into the core of my being, and this affected my self-image during my adolescent development.

I was quick to internalize an emotional focus on my nose more than my other physical characteristics. The negative impact of the word picture planted into my subconscious by Marlie would remain with me throughout my youth. My emotional focus on my physical attributes would overshadow my relationship with my family members.

Marlie can't recall making this comment as a young girl to me; it was years later that I reminded her of the insulting remark. Now, as a grown man, I don't hold anything against Marlie for throwing a negative curveball into my adolescent self-image, which in turn affected my self-esteem.

I was already self-conscious about my nose in particular because I had a bulbous-shaped nose, but Marlie's surprising remarks had caught me completely emotionally off guard. My focus concerning my physical characteristics was brought into acute focus emotionally and mentally by the words spoken by Marlie.

I thank God for helping me to realize that I had natural God-given abilities and talents back then that enabled me to rise above the negative impacts of life that would try to hinder my developmental years.

My father, Benjamin Scone, brought home a good-looking banjo that one of his barber customers was willing to give to me provided I would practice playing the instrument. I would accompany my father on the guitar at church during song worship with only a few banjo chords that my father had taught me. I found that I became irritated whenever my father would ask me if I had practiced that day.

Unfortunately, I never consistently practiced playing the banjo, and in time my father gave the instrument back to his customer. It was a lot more fun to play with my friends, and eventually I would try out for the baseball team as a young boy. My coach and my teammates discovered that I had a strong pitching arm that was pretty effective in striking out the opposing team's batters. I discovered that I enjoyed the competition in the game of baseball, and I became pretty good at it.

I was well liked by my classmates in Cloverdale Elementary School in Clover Valley. I discovered that I was a pretty fast runner, and I enjoyed recess time racing against a friend or competing in playground sports activities. I enjoyed talking with girls whom I liked on the playground too. I also earned quite a reputation for being strong as a fighter, who could whip his opponent primarily as a good wrestler.

I am grateful that I didn't get into a good scrap with a stronger adversary in grade school than my good friend Frank White. Frank fought with me in the front yard of the White family's home, and he put all of his strength into giving me a good whipping.

Even considering Frank's home turf advantage, I was surprised by how strong my friend really was and just how quickly he had moved to get me into a strong wrestling hold that I wasn't able to overcome at my young age. I determined to increase my strength by lifting a suitcase in our family basement that I had put a lot of books into to increase its weight until I was able to purchase my own weight set. I became a strong young boy with real potential for a future in baseball.

I was a skinny boy growing up in Clover Valley, and for some, I came to be known as Skinny Kurtess. I found that I had good strength as a slender, wiry boy, who had earned myself a good reputation among my elementary peers.

I know that many people were surprised that such a skinny child could accomplish such feats of strength that could get others to pay attention. Marlie and I liked to playact in our living room at times; Marlie would fake a punch at me, and I would grab her arm while bending down to lift her up onto my shoulder. I was to show my strength in front of one of our friends or family members by spinning Marlie around, who was now bent over on my shoulder.

I showed my friend Kyle Schurman that I not only was strong, but I had swift boxing capabilities, when we were sparring together in the backyard of the Scone family's residence. Kyle and I were only in the second grade, but I was able to come at Kyle with quick jabbing speed and hard-hitting punching power until Kyle got to the place that he conceded that I was the better at boxing with gloves on.

I remember my brother, Daniel, telling me that being slender has its advantages in karate, a form of martial arts. Daniel told me that someone who was wiry could hurt an opponent in a big way. I have learned that when a martial artist combines speed with being wiry and having focus, he carries tremendous punching power that can cause an adversary critical damage.

I recall a time when I and my friends Frank White and Treat Munson decided that we needed something to sit on in our tree fort. The tree fort was situated in a large maple tree on the north side of the Scone family lot, and it had a solid wood floor with plenty of space to stand up in or to sit down on. What we needed was something to sit down on in the tree fort, so we decided to bring up a large, round stump by rope. We tied the rope securely around the stump and began to pull the heavy stump with the strong, thick rope that the stump was attached to.

Treat and I were doing most of the work of pulling the stump up from the ground directly into the front of the tree fort flooring. As the pulling became more of a struggle, Frank began helping out by adding his strength to the strenuous pulling on the rope. As the three boys were intensely focused on working together to pull up our new tree-fort furniture to add to our home in the big maple tree, we were unaware that the rope had wrapped itself around Frank's leg and foot. When it became obvious that we three were not going to be able to pull the stump up from under the front board of our tree platform without the strength of someone stronger than ourselves, we decided to let the stump fall to the ground. The suddenly taut rope descending quickly to the ground caught Frank's leg and flipped him up in the air as he fell to the ground.

Frank landed flat on his back as Treat and I looked on. Frank wasn't making any movement. He just lay there, but his left hand began to shake from the traumatic impact with the ground. Treat and I climbed down from the tree fort as fast as we could to check on our good friend. To our surprise, thank God, Frank was all right, with no serious injuries. My mother ended up paying for the doctor's bill when he went for his examination.

I was voted to be first lieutenant by popular vote at Cloverdale Elementary School as number one flag patrolman of our crosswalk guard. My friend Joe Daniels was voted captain as the second flag patrolman.

I remember one day while Mr. Nelson was sharing one of his talks with his fifth grade class that I placed my right arm into my left shirtsleeve and I then put my left arm into my right shirtsleeve—just for something to do right in the middle of class. Mr. Nelson was sitting on my desk as he was sharing with the class, and I still had my shirt on at the time. Mr. Nelson liked to share stories with the class to maintain the pupils' attention on various topics that he thought would be of interest to the class. I wasn't able to pull my arms back inside of my shirt and then place my arms back into the correct shirtsleeves. I found myself in a real predicament. Mr. Nelson saw the pickle that I had gotten myself into, and he had me get up in front of the class to show them the difficulty I was in. The class got a real kick out of my predicament that day. I got the attention of my teacher and my classmates, but I never repeated my awkward crisscross shirt episode again in school.

When Mr. Nelson found me chewing my fingernails, he would put adhesive tape on my fingers to help me consciously quit the bad habit. I believe this preventative action by Mr. Nelson helped me be more conscientious about a nervous habit.

I remember a rather effective way my brother Daniel helped me to be conscientious about chewing my food with my mouth closed: Daniel told me that I sounded like I was slopping hogs. Daniel's surprising remark caught me off guard, but it had a profound impact upon the way I ate my food from then on. I became more conscientious about chewing with my mouth closed at the dinner table thanks to my big brother.

One night I was able to have my friend Treat Munson stay overnight so that he could go to church with me that Sunday morning. Treat had poured himself a large bowl of cereal with some cold milk that the Scone family got from the Arthers, who owned milking cows.

If one of their cows happened to eat something unpleasant, it could affect the taste of the milk. The milk had soured, and Treat quickly detected the bad taste. Daniel, being the big tough athlete, came into the kitchen and told Treat to hold his nose and choke it down. Daniel poured himself a large bowl of cereal, took one bite of the bad-tasting breakfast food, and said, "Oh man," while he quickly removed himself from the table. Even my tough big brother, Daniel, couldn't handle the sickening spoiled milk that Sunday morning.

I had eaten my small bowl of cereal with the good-tasting homogenized milk that had been in the refrigerator along with the skim milk without any sour-tasting problems.

One Saturday afternoon, I went to an activity center for boys in Graniteville, across the Sussan River, to check out the club for boys and to see what activities I might be able to take part in. I saw that the club had a ping-pong table and a gymnasium for youth to play basketball in. I didn't have any friends to play with me at the time, so I decided to wander down to the basement area to check it out. I remember there was a large-sized youth who suddenly seized me, took me down onto a wrestling mat, and began aggressively trying to unbuckle my pants belt.

The large boy had caught me completely off guard, and feeling totally defenseless and powerless to resist the overpowering adolescent attacker, I began to cry. The big bully immediately let go of me and quickly took off up the stairs. At the time of the incident, there were no safeguards in place to avoid my attacker. The destructive impact upon me had not left an indelible impression on my person. The suddenness of the attack had left me unharmed bodily, but it had caught me unaware.

Looking back at the situation, I thank the good Lord for His protection against something that could have turned out to be something more sinister.

My brother, Daniel, was a real sports enthusiast, who had taken an interest in my athletic abilities. Daniel worked with me to help me develop good pitching control skills. Daniel's friend Randy also took me under his coaching wing; his good-sized frame provided a larger target to pitch to, which made it easier to hit the catcher's glove. I realize that a pitcher's object is to throw to the catcher's glove regardless of the size of the catcher, but I found it was easier to throw strikes as a young boy by having a larger-sized catcher to catch my fast balls.

I recall Peter Sanders, who was a quality catcher and played for another team, making a remark that I was a faster baseball pitcher than one of the league's best pitchers, Phil Ness. As a boy, it was nice to hear Peter's significant comment emphasizing my dominance as a prestigious fastball pitcher, although the remark had been a surprise to me concerning my pitching speed. I was riding the wave of good success as an outstanding baseball pitcher when I had a disastrous experience on the pitching mound during tournament play.

I had just gotten through pitching my team to a tremendous victory over a really good team, the Aware Repeats, when my coach had me turn around and immediately start the next tournament game. It was early in the second game that I threw my arm out pitching at the age of twelve due to ligament muscle strain; it had been an unfortunate bad call by my coach. It became the last game of the baseball season for me, and this turned out to be a good thing because my injured arm needed plenty of time to rest from pitching.

I participated in playing basketball with a Clover Valley elementary team, but I found that I was not as good a basketball player as my older brother, Daniel, was. One day I had quickly taken the basketball down the St. Paul's Catholic School gymnasium floor, and I made a fantastic jump shot that cleared the hoop with a swish. The only problem with my perfect basket was that I had added to the other team's score. I eventually tried out as a freshman for the Clover Valley High School basketball team, but I found myself getting cut from the tryouts. I was disappointed that I wasn't considered good enough to play on the junior varsity basketball team for the high school, but looking back, I understand the good reason was that I lacked the fundamental basic skills to be a really good player, who could be seen as a major contributor to the team. I remember a quote from my brother, Daniel: "You can't put in what God has left out." I realize that I wasn't gifted by God with the talents and skills to play the game of basketball as other athletes have been given in this life, such as Michael Jordan.

I tried out for the Clover Valley High School football team in my freshman year, and I successfully made the team. I managed to get into one game, and the play called for me to go out for a pass. Unfortunately for me, I never got to touch the football. It was a night game and I was able to see the football flying in the night air, but I lost sight of it and it went sailing over my head onto the field. I wasn't the most outstanding football player anyway, and I didn't care to watch the games from the sidelines. I wasn't interested in trying to stay warm on those cold winter nights, but I continued to attend the team's practices and watch the games as a spectator player from the sidelines or talk to a friend on the sidelines while the games were in play or during halftime. I never tried out for the football team again after my freshman year as a Clover Valley Lion.

I had inherited the Scone nose, as my father had from Grandfather Scone. The Scone nose was definitely more prominent and exaggerated than the nose on my mother's side of the family. When I began attending school, I enjoyed talking with girls at an early age. I discovered that certain girls took an interest in talking to me too. The girls didn't seem to have a problem with my outward appearance based on their interactions with me.

My brother, Daniel, had taken a serious interest in sports, and he became extremely good in track and basketball. I had already become a pretty good baseball pitcher in grade school, and I continued pitching into my junior high and high school years after my arm was healed by the Lord. Playing sports had given me a healthy external perspective about life as a team player. However, my introverted self-consciousness concerning my nose was a very sensitive subject matter.

One day I was playing football on the Clover Valley Lions' baseball field. I called out, "Big play, big play," before the play began. One of my high school classmates called out, "Big nose." This insensitive remark caused me to shut down emotionally, and I remained subdued during the remainder of our football game. I had concluded early in my life that if anyone made an unkind remark concerning my nose or made fun of my appearance, I would not trust that person to be one of my friends. That clearly became my relationship rule for life to protect myself from negative perceptions regarding my physical appearance.

My father, Benjamin Scone, was a conscientious pastor at the Lupine Assembly of God Church. He desired to see souls saved and be filled by the blessed Holy Spirit with power. He barbered in Clover Valley, and another time in Graniteville Heights to help put food on the table and meet his family's needs.

My mother, Jessica, worked faithfully along with my father in the ministry to prepare Christians to live for the Lord Jesus Christ. Benjamin was extremely self-conscious and introverted as a pastor of the church. It took a lot of courage on his part to stand up in front of the congregation to preach and teach to them.

I had my own bouts with self-consciousness about my prominent nose. It was clearly visible for all to see whether I was in church, at school, or playing baseball in front of crowds of supporting fans at the various baseball fields in Clover Valley and Graniteville.

Playing baseball helped me to focus my attention on hitting the catcher's glove, striking out the batters, or allowing my fielders to throw out an advancing base runner. Since baseball is a team sport, I came to realize that every player on the team has a very important role to play in helping the team to win.

I enjoyed playing at Colfax, in the Pacific Northwest, in McNeil's baseball stadium against a really good team from Spokane. The baseball stadium had a wooden fence surrounding the ball field, which we weren't accustomed to playing on. When I began warming up on the pitching mound, I heard one of the Spokane batters offer advice to the leadoff hitter that he needed to swing faster.

After I heard the good advice to the leadoff batter, I reared back and began throwing even harder to the catcher's glove. I felt a strong need to demonstrate that I was a dominating fastball thrower, and I wanted to provide the opposing hitters a really big show of pure power pitching.

I pitched for three innings without giving up any runs, and then the coach called for a pitching change. Coaches had a rule where they would call for a pitching change just to prevent damaging a young boy's arm during the games. First baseman Carl Davidson pitched for the last three innings of the game.

I scored on a base hit by Carl, and our team went on to win three to two. It was an exciting game to play in because the opposing team's pitcher and catcher were sons of the female coach, and they were on the top team from Spokane.

The mighty victory built up my confidence that I had what it took to help my team win big games. My good friend Bud, aka "Brutus Knuckles," from Lincoln, Arkansas, thought it was interesting when he heard about the exciting developments of the game: I had pitched three innings without giving up a run, first baseman Carl then pitched the last three innings and gave up two runs, and we all obviously realized the importance of playing with intensity and all the healthy competition that took place during the summer game, which happened to turn out in my team's favor. The team had something to celebrate knowing we had triumphed over, and defeated, a really good team from Spokane.

I recall an important game during which I was to pitch against a strong left-handed pitcher named Gene Bradshaw at the Clover Valley High School baseball field. Gene had good speed and excellent control that I and my teammates, the Little Aces baseball team, hadn't faced before.

The Ultimate Violation

I gave up one unfortunate hard-earned run in the first inning, and then I found myself really bearing down on doing my best to mow down the batting opposition of the Meadowlarks baseball team during the rest of the game.

The tall, lanky, hard-throwing Gene Bradshaw had given up a walk to my teammate Doug Seltzer, who played first base for the Little Aces. Gene was closely watching Doug moving back and forth off of first base when he glanced toward the catcher in his side wind-up position. Gene saw Doug take a large lead off the first base bag, challenging him to pick him off first base. Doug was preparing to take off and steal second base when Gene suddenly threw a quick throw to his first baseman. Doug made a valiant effort to get back to first base before he could be tagged out, but it was too late. Doug was called out by the umpire.

Doug was our only base runner in a good position to potentially score a run for us, and it was a costly out that the Little Aces couldn't seem to recover from. I went on to shut down the Meadowlarks baseball team from scoring any more stinging runs against me, but the one-to-nothing loss was certainly a disappointing game that I would not like to repeat again anytime soon. I hoped that my team had a good chance of winning the next game should the two teams ever get to play again, but I positively didn't like the agony of defeat, which the Little Aces weren't accustomed to experiencing. I came to recognize that there were a number of excellent pitchers playing for other teams in Clover Valley who could give the Little Aces baseball team a tough challenge on any good day.

I fully know that life is a reflection of how we feel about ourselves. I have discovered that a person's life consists of a lot more than the abundance of things that we possess, especially when our lives are not totally wrapped up in our physical appearance.

The world's standards for being accepted and a true success in life require that one have brains, beauty, and bucks. This standard of measurement has a strong influence in the world on one's ability to get ahead in certain success-oriented businesses, political arenas, friendships and relationships, talent contests, arts and theaters, and the movies, as well as on whether one may get promoted to a leadership position in a good Christian church. This is not God's standard for the pathway to receive promotions in any walk of life. I now realize that man looks on the outward appearance, but God looks at the heart of men and women regarding their motives for life's pursuits.

39

Having good character is worth a lot more than pursuing our own self-interests at the neglect and expense of others on the pathway to successful living. People have their own idea of what makes them feel good about themselves, and having good looks can definitely help along the course of life. It is important to note that adolescents who have a favorable view of themselves in relation to their looks will generally be more stable in their self-concepts of themselves.

We need to have a positive attitude toward ourselves apart from our self-conscious feelings concerning our outward appearance. If somebody does not believe that God has truly smiled upon him or her with natural physical beauty, I want to encourage the reader with good news. I wasn't the most physically good-looking young boy according to the world's standards either, but I know that God forever loves me and that He expects me to develop other talents for His eternal purposes with God's help. God's love is extended to all.

I appreciate the good times that my family and I enjoyed while doing things together. I remember going on camping trips and fishing with my parents, who were thoughtful, considerate, and willing to reward us children with good times in the great outdoors.

I recall going to Chatcolet Lake, which is a part of the large Coeur d' Alane Lake in the Pacific Northwest, with my family.

I recall fishing off of the dock and the good experience of going out on the lake in a motorboat. My father was good at catching bass at Rocky Point on Coeur d' Alane Lake. My sister Marlie and my brother, Daniel, knew how to catch trout, perch, crappie, and catfish. I wasn't as good at fishing as the rest of my family were, and I wasn't interested in spending a lot of time trying to catch fish.

While other family members were serious about catching fish, I would look for ways to have fun by throwing rocks at birds, hoping to catch a squirrel or chipmunk, playing in the sand, and later when I grew up, trying to bag a bird, squirrel, or chipmunk with my father's long-barrel Remington twenty-two rifle. I found that there are a lot of ways to have fun in the great outdoors.

I enjoyed taking a friend along on one of the family campouts or on one of our great outdoor outings. It was healthy fun just to get out of town on occasion and be able to go up to the mountains or to a nice lake.

I enjoyed the adventure of doing outdoor activities with a good friend more than hanging out with the family all the time. I remember going huckleberry picking in the mountains, which my parents had enjoyed as a traditional activity for years. I wasn't big on picking huckleberries all day on Bald Mountain or any one of the other berry-picking sites, but I enjoyed eating them by themselves and also in a pie that my mother would bake. I have come to appreciate my mom and dad for all of the neat things they were willing and able to do for me and my siblings in order to give us kids a wonderful respect and appreciation for God's pleasurable creation.

I remember going to the A & W root-beer stand in Clover Valley after the family came home from church. I also recall going to the Linguini Restaurant on the outskirts of Graniteville for an enjoyable spaghetti and meatballs with the delicious chicken dinner that was a special treat for the Scone family on a Sunday afternoon after the morning service.

I enjoyed going to the Graniteville rodeo with the Scone family when I was a boy to watch all the exciting rodeo events. I also recall how the family took an interest in coming home Sunday evenings after church, looking forward to watching *The Fugitive* on television.

There were good times in the Scone family as we did things together. I recall coming home one Sunday evening after attending a Christian church service and watching a movie about the life of Christ. I remember crying when I saw them crucify the Lord Jesus on the cross of Calvary. It was a tender moment for me as a young boy to consider the power of an event that I didn't fully understand at the time; I later would come to a greater understanding of the magnitude of God's great love for myself and for all of humanity.

I recall how the Scone family would drive up to Blue Mountain Springs, south of Clover Valley, to do some sledding together. This turned out to be a great winter activity that the entire family enjoyed doing as a group. Putting wax on the hard metal blades helped the sled to slide effortlessly down the white-blanketed sled run.

I liked to get up on the back of my big brother, Daniel, or my father, Benjamin, to make the long run on a fast-moving sled down the snow-covered mountain road to the bottom of the hill. Then we had to make the long trek back up to the top of our sledding slope. I didn't especially appreciate this part of our sledding adventure as a family. I remember different family members using our wooden toboggan prepared by waxing its bottom to get the most speed possible down the long hill road.

I reflect back to another Scone family sledding experience when I got too close to the fire with my rubber boots. I wasn't paying attention to just how near my galoshes were to the hot campfire that the family was enjoying to stay warm on a cold winter's night. My mother, Jessica, happened to catch sight of my boot tips being burned by the heat from the campfire. I needed someone to carefully watch out for my careless actions when I was an innocent child.

As I grew older, I enjoyed making the fast sled run by myself. I found that I needed to stay focused on what I was doing all the way to the bottom of the hill to have a successful sledding experience.

Life was good for me, although the Scone family was not financially classified in the upper crust of society's economic elite. I had heard that the upper crust were a lot of crumbs stuck together with a lot of dough.

The Scone family was not economically rich according to the total income that my mom and dad declared on their income tax form at the end of the year. But the family was rich in talents and abilities, especially when it came to the family's godly Christian heritage. I remember how my family would have Bible devotions together, followed by a time of prayer. I remember how I would want to get together with a friend on a Saturday morning, and yet I was required to spend time with my family and God first. As a young boy, I always wanted to get our devotional time over as quickly as possible.

I liked reading Psalm 117 as a boy because it was the shortest chapter in the Bible. My parents saw that it was necessary to honor God by having someone in our immediate family read a passage from the Word of God and take time for prayer before we left for the day. I now can see that this traditional practice to remember God and His goodness was good for the Scone family.

I remember how my father, brother Daniel, and I enjoyed watching television together. We would really get a hearty laugh out of watching *The Munsters* half-hour program, and how family members took such an interest in watching *The Andy Griffith Program*. These shows seemed to have good, wholesome, family entertainment that either struck a humorous chord in our hearts, had a good family theme, or had a good subject matter that held our interest throughout each program. We had some good times of hearty laughter getting a kick out of watching together the comedy programs.

My father and I seemed to have similar senses of humor, which helped us bond together, especially in our adult years. We could find ourselves laughing together whether my father was giving me a haircut or we were sitting around talking in the house. We could especially have good times as a family together when we incorporated humor into the family relationships. I liked to be funny, telling jokes, and I enjoyed making my family and friends laugh every chance I got.

I found that I could make friends easily by the way I would take an interest in others and show that I really liked being with other people. I also discovered that I could get certain friends to do things with me and for me—like the time that my parents wanted me to help dig out our dirt basement. I was able to get some of my friends to help me dig and empty the dirt out of the wheelbarrow into our large side lot. I was able to hire my friends' help for twenty-five cents an hour for a while before they grew tired of the project. My friends eventually decided to use their time watching television instead of using their time helping me finish the project.

My friendship with my friends couldn't spark any acceptable incentive apart from a raise in pay. They wanted a pay raise to seventy-five cents an hour. I found myself, my brother Daniel, and another hired hand my parents paid were the only ones willing to do the rest of the project. My mom and dad awarded me with a Kawasaki 100 motorcycle as a reward for all of my hard work in completing the digging out of the house basement project. I enjoyed riding my new motorcycle in town, and also when I rode the combo street and dirt bike on gravel roads or dirt trails up Feather Creek south of Clover Valley.

I experienced a life-changing transformation at the mature age of fourteen. I had a personal encounter with Jesus Christ of Nazareth through the transforming person of the Holy Spirit, the Spirit of Christ. My father and mother were between pastorates of a Christian church, and we began attending Clover Valley Assembly of God Church. I remember that Senior Pastor Neal Adams at the Clover Valley Assembly wanted the congregation to have a time of prayer before we left the church that Sunday afternoon.

I remember that as I knelt down for a time of prayer, I sensed a warm presence come over me, which caused me to realize that I needed to invite Jesus Christ to come into my heart and ask His forgiveness for my sins. My new birth experience brought a transforming change into my life, which made a wonderful difference in my thinking, actions, and personal relationship with God and with others. God had made a new person out of me, and I wanted my friends and other non-Christians to come to know Jesus as He had so marvelously revealed Himself to me.

I found that I was becoming excited about the things of God, and I looked forward to reading my Bible when I would come home from school. I discovered that Jesus Christ had produced a newfound meaning into my life and a reason for living. I now looked forward to going to church and sharing my faith with others. Jesus had made a profound change in my life, but I found that not everyone at school was freely willing and wanting to come to Christ Jesus as I had. I remember sharing my testimony about how God had changed my life with a friend postgraduation.

My friend Sidney commented on when he had visually observed the change in my life at the pivotal moment right between my eighth and ninth grades. I told Sidney that he was correct in his recollection as to the exact time when Jesus had wrought a wonderful change in my life. God was doing a good work in my personality, and He would continue to develop godly character into my life. My existence in life would never be the same. Now I would have a friend that sticks closer than a brother living in my heart, and life for all of eternity. My life was now marked by my Creator for God's glory and purposes.

I have learned that my new life in Christ Jesus is to reflect the life and light of God to the people of the world. Jesus is the light of the world, and when He comes into a person's life, He manifests Himself to that individual who willingly loves Him. He then wants that individual to reflect His divine life and light to everyone who does not know Him in a personal way. He is not willing that anyone should be lost; He wants all to come to the knowledge of the truth in Him and the finished work of His cross. The devil wants to extinguish the light and life of Jesus shining out to every person who needs eternal life through Christ Jesus. Satan, the Bible says, comes to steal, kill, and destroy, but "Jesus Christ came that you might have life and have it more abundantly" (John 10:10).

Unfortunately, Satan uses people to seek to extinguish the life and light from a Christian's heart and life through all types of tactics or methods. The Bible is the Word of God, and His glorious promises will keep the reader from sin—or sin will keep the reader from walking and living in the light of His Word.

I recognize that the Lord's divine presence is reaching out to people as they sincerely call upon His glorious name in spirit and in truth.

Nothing that this world has to offer compares to a person who has come to experience eternal life in Christ Jesus our Lord.

I appreciate how my brother, Daniel, was good about encouraging me to improve myself in baseball and other athletic abilities. Daniel shared with me about one man who was able to do six thousand push-ups which I understood to mean consecutively six thousand at a single block of time. For a number of weeks, I had been doing my push-ups and sit ups to keep myself in good physical shape, and mentally preparing myself for the physical challenge I was thinking of participating in. I decided to work on my own physical conditioning, and one night I was able to do 395 push-ups without putting my knees down to rest. This tremendous physical feat caused me to work up a good sweat roughly within an hour because I paused and resumed my push-ups a number of times to meet my goal. I had determined to persevere until I reached my predetermined goal of the highest number of push-ups for myself during one single block of time.

I didn't have a professional physical trainer hovering over me with a stop watch during my rigorous challenging feat of endurance.

I found that my chest and arm muscles were larger and were harder from doing the high number of push-ups. I was interested in muscle tone and definition for my arms and chest, but I was not interested in becoming muscle-bound, which might give me pitching difficulties in the future. I decided against pursuing a goal of increasing the number of push-ups I could physically do roughly in an hour because I hoped to pitch baseball for a major league team someday if I were physically capable and everything worked out just right for me to play in the major leagues.

I discovered that I had a good deal of confidence acting in front of people. One night at the Graniteville Assembly of God Church, I was willing to participate in a church play. I was boldly able to say my actor's lines and then pour milk upon another actor's head. I discovered that the audience laughed at my performance.

I was delighted to know that I had pleased the audience. One day at school, I starred as a Daniel Boone character and put my friend over my shoulder to present myself as a mighty frontiersman who had bagged myself a bear. I discovered that I had God-given abilities that I understand now only needed to be developed by consistent effort and use.

Daniel Scone took karate lessons, and he was able to compete against a martial arts opponent and decisively defeat him. He went on to receive his master's in athletic administration, and he has become a very successful coach.

I have become pretty good in ping-pong, baseball, and picking on my five-string Deering banjo. It took a lot of practice to become good at each individual hobby or art.

I didn't receive the most prestigious grades in my elementary, junior high, and senior high school years. I later discovered that I had a good memory for details and for memorizing dialogues in school. I did receive extra credit for my memory skills in college later as an adult, and I received good grades while attending Union's Theology Institute.

When I read the six ways to make people like you in the book *How to Win Friends and Influence People* by Dale Carnegie, this positively influenced me to reach out and make friends with a lot of people.

I was motivated to make friends with good-quality people, and Dale had provided me with some good tools to work with that provided the right way to go about making friends. I wanted to reach out to others at Clover Valley High School because I had a friendly nature about me, but I desired to be friendly in a positive way for the cause of Christ Jesus because I wanted to influence young people in my school to come to know the giver of salvation and eternal life.

I was awarded a significant honor by the high school seniors at Clover Valley High School. I give all the credit to my personal Lord and Savior Jesus Christ for this significant award that my classmates kindly bestowed upon me. I also won a clock radio, which was given to me from a drawing they had at the senior prom dance for the graduates.

I recall one significant moment in time when my personal Lord and Savior helped me during an important baseball game. I was pitching for the Granite-Clover Valley Basic Legion baseball team when I barely missed the plate with a rock-solid fastball called a ball by the umpire. The pitch missed the outside corner of the plate, and I found myself using a four-letter swear word softly that only I could hear while standing out on the mound.

You can hear this barnyard word blared out by an angry rancher on any given day. I was certainly disappointed with myself for not throwing the pitch across the plate. I took time to whisper a prayer to the Lord to forgive me for this momentary transgression; I was not accustomed to using profanity on the ball field or anywhere else. I realized that I played baseball with non-Christians, but I had never taken on their bad habits of using profanity whenever they would become angry or extremely frustrated by their on-the-field errors or mistakes.

The Lord forgave me for saying an objectionable swear word that day, and I have not had another problem with uttering profanity during an angry or frustrating moment in my life ever again. God helped me to be conscious of the words that I spoke in His presence and in the presence of other people.

I was a compliant and obedient child growing up in the Scone family home. My parents, Benjamin and Jessica, didn't have any ongoing disciplinary problems in raising me since I had a sensitive conscience and an easygoing disposition during my developmental adolescent years.

I recall one night that my father, Benjamin, had a talk with his four children regarding something that he was not happy about that was happening in the home. Since I was just a young boy at the time, I don't recollect what my father was talking about that night; but I remember that after our father had taken time to communicate his displeasure with his children, he took the belt and gave Carol and Daniel a good spanking for what he felt they had done wrong.

I recall that Marlie stood up afterward and said she thought that she also deserved a spanking. Benjamin complied by giving her a licking with the belt as well.

I remember that I remained sitting down and never volunteered to have my bottom spanked for what my father considered bad behavior. I recall that there were times that I needed to be disciplined for misbehavior during my growing-up years. My mother, Jessica, usually did the disciplining with a lilac switch to my legs and bottom in the Scone family home.

Jessica would ask me to go out and break off a lilac stem for her to use on me. I would typically pick out a thin, flimsy lilac stem instead of a thick one that could hold up for a number of lashings. The spankings generally were short this way and soon forgotten, without any serious lasting pain.

The comparison between my nose and my brother's was made evident one day by Daniel's wife Allison's revealing comment that my nose was more exaggerated than Daniel's nose. After Allison made the surprising remark, Daniel tried to soften the negative impact of her insensitive comment, although her evaluation was accurate according to any physical comparison between the brothers' noses.

Daniel quickly commented that I had a better personality than he had.

I made a mental note of Allison's evaluation concerning my nose compared to Daniel's, but I never tried to counter what she had to say at the time nor since.

I allowed people to say what they felt like saying concerning my physical characteristics, but I didn't try to retaliate by making critical remarks about their physical features in return. I realized the subject matter was too emotionally charged to get into negative mudslinging about physical characteristics that God had created and that were out of my control to change anyway.

I knew that my prominent nose was physically not as attractive as my brother Daniel's was, but I was not constantly mentally and emotionally focused on my physical characteristics.

I had learned and adopted a saying as to what true optimism is: "True optimism is having the cheerful frame of mind that enables a teakettle to sing though in hot water up to its nose." I endeavored to apply a consistent positive and optimistic attitude toward life, even in the face of adverse conditions, circumstances, and negative-thinking people.

Daniel had married his lovely bride, Allison, when he was twenty-five years old, I was asked by my brother to be his best man. Naturally, I was willing to be Daniel's best man. Daniel and Allison have been married for twenty-seven years. God has blessed Daniel and Allison throughout the years in holy matrimony, and they have four talented children.

One day my girlfriend Cindy and I planned to meet up with my parents at Priest Lake, northeast of Spokane. Cindy and I went into the Priest Lake Restaurant to use the restroom facilities before meeting with my parents. I found that the men's room had water on the floor, and this had left moisture on the toilet seat. I laid toilet tissue on the seat cover before sitting down. When I came out of the bathroom, I didn't realize that I had toilet tissue sticking out of my pants. I noticed how friendly everyone seemed toward me; everyone had a smile on their face when they saw me or when they talked with me. The good people seemed to really enjoy having me there. One man took a real interest in my inquiry about the bears that had been sighted at a specific northern point of the lake.

When Cindy and I left to go out to my car, I came to the self-conscious realization that I had toilet tissue stuck to my backside. I now realized the reason why everyone had been so friendly with me inside the restaurant. I told Cindy, "Let's get out of here." I was too embarrassed to show my face around the Priest Lake Restaurant any longer. I want the reader to know that these are the facts regarding the situation that had taken place in the restaurant; I see this as one of the most embarrassing moments in my life.

My life-changing experience had given me the confidence that I needed in life. I discovered that whenever I took time to pray about a situation that I was facing, God would come through and answer my prayers. I remember one particular time when I couldn't find my contact lens; I thought for certain it had fallen onto the floor. I searched diligently by looking in all the obvious places, and even looking on top of my bedroom dresser. It was nowhere to be found. I then asked the Lord to help me find my contact lens. I immediately got the idea to look inside of my dresser drawer. I could see that my dresser top had an inch or two overhang, and it seemed a total impossibility for my contact lens to ever end up in the drawer. I decided to go ahead and look inside the drawer anyway. To my great surprise, my contact lens was inside of the dresser drawer. There was another time when the Lord helped me to find my contact lens, which had fallen onto the sawdust floor at the Crest Forest Industries sawmill I worked at in Graniteville.

The Lord was showing me that He was interested in the little things and the big things in my life.

God continued to answer my prayers, and He would continue to be faithful, good, and kind to me throughout my adolescent years.

From Adolescence to Adulthood

When I invited the Lord Jesus Christ into my heart and life at the tender age of fourteen, I found that my new life in Christ had become the best decision I had ever made. Jesus Christ changed me into a new creature in Christ, and I wanted my friends to come to know the one true God, as I had.

I would come home with my schoolbooks in my arms only to end up setting them aside to spend time reading the Holy Bible. The Word of God was doing a new work in my life, and this life-changing experience was making a profound difference in my relationships with others.

I remember one important day when I had to make a choice for Christ that would forever change my relationship with some good friends of mine. I and three of my good friends were on our way to the Lion's Den in Clover Valley for a school dance. We were walking over to the Lion's Den, where high school teenagers would gather to dance while the live rock bands performed on stage, when I made a decision to hold up before crossing Main Street, allowing my friends to continue their journey to the Den.

I had come to a crossroads in my life: I needed to leave the world's interests and activities behind me, and take a firm stand for Christ Jesus, my Lord and Savior.

I felt within myself that I had to take a stand for the Lord if I was going to live for God. Without telling my friends that I needed to go home that night, I turned around and walked back home, recognizing I had made the right decision.

I found that my decision not to continue on to the Lion's Den strongly affected my relationship with my good friends. I found that people I had considered to be good friends were now cold toward me, but I knew within myself that I had made the right decision in life.

Reflecting back on my decision for Christ Jesus, I only wish now that I had had the good sense to sufficiently communicate to my friends that I needed to go home because I didn't feel right about going to the Lion's Den that night. Even if my friends hadn't understood my decision to return home, it would have been the appropriate thing for me to do to keep my friends from cooling off toward me.

I was a young Christian, and being a teenager, I didn't know the best way to use wisdom in dealing with my friends who still wanted to maintain a friendship with the world. I learned that my friends would go to beer parties at times, where they had kegs of beer to drink; I didn't want to have any association with the beer drinking.

My family believed in traditional family values, and drinking alcohol was not part of my family cultural experience. The Bible and my Christian church warned me about making friendship with the world and not to be a partaker with the things in the world, which included drinking alcohol in excess. I was doing my best to make wise choices to avoid the evils in the world that could be destructive to my walk with Christ.

The Bible says:

> Do not be unequally yoked together with unbelievers. For what fellowship has righteousness with lawlessness? And what communion has light with darkness? And what accord has Christ with Belial? Or what part has a believer with an unbeliever? And what agreement has the temple of God with idols? For you are the temple of the living God.

As God has said:

> "I will dwell in them And walk among them. I will be their God, And they shall be my people."
>
> Therefore "Come out from among them And be separate," says the Lord. "Do not touch what is unclean, And I will receive you."
>
> "I will be a Father to you, And you shall be My sons and daughters," says the Lord Almighty.
>
> Therefore, having these promises, beloved, let us cleanse ourselves from all filthiness of the flesh and spirit, perfecting

holiness in the fear of God. (2 Cor. 6:14-18; . . . 2 Cor. 7:1 NKJV).

I wanted to maintain my relationship with my Savior and still be able to participate in good wholesome activities with my friends. I wanted to be able to play baseball and ping-pong with them, play over-the-line, go bowling, or attend one of Daniel's Clover Valley Lions' basketball games. I enjoyed playing miniature golf and tennis, and getting together for bites to eat. Another activity I participated in was scuba diving with my friend Kevin and his dad up the Big Rock River; we also did some scuba diving together across from the Crest Forest Industries Mill in Graniteville. I remember reaching out to touch a large fish in the Big Rock River, when it made a sudden turn and came right at us. Kevin began to laugh, and he needed to make a quick rise to the surface when I witnessed the large-scaled creature seemingly on the attack. I realized it was trying to escape from possibly becoming dinner to a larger creature reaching out to touch it.

When my friends and I wanted to get together for good times, the key word was Brazos. I had learned that call word to come together for something important from watching the *Over-the-Hill Gang* movie: the captain summoned the Texas Rangers, who—although now old senior citizens—when called upon for duty, came together to take care of some important business by handling outlaws to the best of their abilities.

I and my three good friends Kevin, David, and Scott saw our getting together as something important, with a lot of good fun times together. We recognized that our coming together was something big and exciting, something to look forward to because we had something significant to do or to take care of that we considered important.

My three friends and I were talented athletes, and we all played together on the Clover Valley High School baseball team. Being involved in sports had helped to bring about our friendship, and we enjoyed getting together whenever we could.

I remained friendly with my good friends although I wasn't as close with them as I had been before my Christian conversion. The Lord had brought about a significant change for the better in my heart and life, and as I continued to grow in the grace and knowledge of the Lord Jesus Christ, God continued to help me through the good times and the difficult times that I would face in life.

One summer, Kevin, David, Scott, and I decided to camp out at Buck State Park. I remember how we were enjoying our campout by having dinner together around a nice cozy fire followed by playing cards inside the tent, with Kevin's kerosene lantern providing good lighting for our game. The four of us had a grand time being together again like old times.

The following day, after having cereal for breakfast, Kevin and I decided to build a rock pathway across Feather Creek by dropping rocks into the swift-flowing creek. I positioned my hard-toed boots securely onto a rock sticking up in the creek.

I put my hands out for Kevin to drop a large rock onto them for me to toss it into the creek to the left of my position. When Kevin heard the go-ahead from me, he dropped the big rock. The rock went right through my hands and landed squarely on my right foot. The boot I was wearing hadn't protected me when the rock slammed down. I suddenly felt intense pain in my right foot like I had never felt before.

The acute pain I was feeling in my right foot caused me not to care about getting wet—I walked right through the creek to sit down on some smaller rocks situated on the creek bed.

As I was hurting from the pain in my foot, I looked down at the rocks and observed a spider walking along on the creek bed.

I suddenly felt like throwing up when my friend David inquired if I wanted him to build a fire. I didn't care to have a fire built for me as I threw up on the rocks from the sheer trauma of my painful experience.

I saw Kevin and David smiling about the situation, not knowing the full agonizing pain that I was in. David and Scott helped to carry me back to the tent, where I was able to get some rest. I was able to get some sleep before I was awakened by my three friends rolling rocks down the hill into Feather Creek. The sleep helped immeasurably to relieve my pain, since we had no pain medication on the campout.

When it came time to leave the park, my friends carried me by taking turns two at a time crossing their arms together to provide a carrying seat for me down the gravel Feather Creek Road. After my good friends had carried me for less than a mile, a truck stopped and ended up providing transportation for the four of us all the way into Clover Valley Heights to Kevin's house.

We were blessed to have been given a ride at that crucial time; with my foot seriously hurt, I might not have been able to get back home.

Upon arriving at Kevin's house, I finally removed my boot and sock. To my surprise, my foot and toes were swollen and black and blue.

Kevin's dad gave me a ride home, which I appreciated. When it came time for me to have my foot X-rayed by the doctor, I learned that I had broken my big right toe, and the two toes next to it were fractured with hairline cracks. I had to use crutches for a while going to Clover Valley High School, but I eventually recovered without having to have a cast put on any of my toes. I am grateful that I don't experience any residual pain from any of my toes that were hurt during the rock-dropping incident at Feather Creek.

I am grateful for my good friends who took the time to help a friend in need. When my big toe was broken that unfortunate day, I was in a world of hurt. I appreciate having friends who care when you're hurting in the worst kind of way. I understand by firsthand experience that a friend who helps a good friend in need is a good friend indeed.

I remember a powerful evangelist, Dwayne Friend, who strongly influenced my walk with Christ as a young believer. I would come home after a Sunday night church service to find my father watching Dwayne Friend preaching a sermon on television. My life was positively impacted by the powerful teaching of this spiritually stimulating Christian evangelist.

One day my mother, Jessica, and my father, Benjamin, drove over to Colfax to hear Dwayne Friend preach an exciting sermon at an evangelistic crusade. After they returned home, they told me that they had gone to hear Dwayne Friend preach. The next day, I was able to go with my parents to hear the Christian evangelist myself and enjoy the powerful crusade service. After the wonderful service, I had the golden opportunity to talk with Dwayne Friend. I remember how Dwayne shared with me how to walk with Christ. He said that God had a million doors for me to walk through, and if I found those doors, I would truly know what life was about. My personal encounter with Dwayne Friend that eventful day would make a profound difference in my life for years to come.

I discovered at the age of fifteen that I felt that the Lord had given to me a pastor's heart. I found that I cared about people's souls and their eternal destinies in the future. The Bible tells us that Jesus saw people as sheep without a shepherd, needing salvation.

I have come to the realization that human souls need to have a spiritual guide to help lead them safely through this life. I have come to see that the Lord Jesus Christ is the good Shepherd, and He, through the power of the Holy Spirit, wants to protect us from all harmful predators in this life. Christians need to be aware that they need to guard their hearts and govern their lives for the Lord's work. People, like sheep, are easily led astray by ravenous wolves disguised as sheep; good Christians can be misled just as well by the big bad wolf, which doesn't care about the sheep nor their individual interests.

The family united acts as a shelter, a shield, and protection to protect each family member from being hurt by wolves in the world who want to hurt the sheep for their own selfish interests and pursuits.

I would like to keep people from being hurt, used, and abused by individuals under the control of the evil one. We all must stay alert to the wolves that diligently look for souls who are alone without any protection.

When I was fifteen, Kevin, David, Scott, and I decided that we wanted to go swimming in the Clover Valley swimming pool late at night. The swimming pool had been closed for hours when we climbed over the wire fence in order to take a swim in the refreshing, cool water.

I had taken my underwear and socks off and placed them into a brown paper sack before getting into the chlorine-filled pool. All four of us took off our shirts and shoes, and spent a good amount of time in the pool before leaving into the dark night air. When we climbed back over the fence that warm summer night, we walked together across the Clover Valley baseball and football fields. We crossed over Main Street and entered the west side of River View Park, doing our level best to stay out of sight from any headlights of vehicles that we might spot. We got about halfway into the city park before we saw a car coming up the alley across Sorrel Avenue on the north side of the park. We tried to avoid being spotted, but when we saw the vehicle make a sudden turn, we knew that we had been detected by the occupants in the fast-moving automobile.

I ran as fast as I could with my friend David across the park and across Seventh Street into the driveway of Marvel's Funeral Home. Kevin and Scott jumped over a concrete wall into the yard of a home on the south side of the funeral home. David and I found that the car we first saw on the north side of the city park was heading in the same direction that we were going as fast as we could run.

David and I found ourselves running through Marvel's Funeral Home parking lot and then making a quick turn south up the alleyway. Every turn that we made, the car with its bright headlights and noisy muffler came speeding right behind us.

We were looking for a backyard that we might be able to quickly dash into, but all I saw was the back of fences all along the narrow alley between home after home. David managed to find an opening leading to a backyard of one home that I had missed seeing. With the fast car hot on my heels, I decided to hold up, for it seemed I had been caught by someone who had taken a real unsolicited interest in me. When I turned around after stopping my hasty run, I observed that it was a Clover Valley police car that had pursued us.

The police officer wanted to check my paper sack, with my underwear and socks still inside. While I was being detained momentarily by the officer, my friends were looking on through the fences in the alleyway.

I got a free ride in the police car to the Clover Valley Police Station for breaking curfew as a minor. When my father, Benjamin, was contacted to come pick up his delinquent son at the police department, he had been sleeping in his comfortable bed. Benjamin signed the release papers and drove me back to our home.

As we were heading home, I discovered that my dad was pretty cool about the whole thing. Benjamin had remarked to me when he saw another vehicle pulled over by a police car with its lights flashing, "Don't they have anything else better to do?"

I discovered as an adult that not all was good in the Scone family even after I had gloriously met the Lord. I learned that the man, Randell Wikum, who married my oldest sister, Carol, had molested my sister Marlie when she was just a teenager. Marlie didn't know how to deal with the horrible pain and guilt from Randell's molestation. Marlie began acting out sinful behaviors in her relationships with the men she dated. Marlie had gotten involved with drugs and alcohol as a teenager, and there were many times that she didn't go to school during the day.

Daniel thought Marlie was faking it when she would choose to stay home from school so often. He didn't know how Marlie had been horribly hurt from the molestation by Randell.

I observed different behaviors in Marlie's attitude and life, but being a teenager, I didn't realize at the time that the best thing that I could do for her was to pray for her to be set free and healed by Christ Jesus, and to have others continue to pray that the Lord would make a significant difference in her life for time and eternity. She would also need the tender healing touch of our gracious Lord Jesus Christ in her heart, mind, and emotions.

I discovered years later that Randell considered himself to be a self-made man and thought highly of himself. Randell also considered himself to be God's gift to women. Throughout his marriage to Carol, he was an unfaithful philanderer and had affairs with different women. Randell had even tried to come onto Daniel's wife, Allison, with his seductive ways early on in their marriage. I never heard any specific details exactly what Randell had done to or with Allison, but apparently she had felt uncomfortable by his actions or words, which were inappropriate for a young married woman to experience or encounter coming from a married man. Randell was a charmer with the ladies, and he was worldly-wise in how to win women for his own self interests. Randell served four years with the navy, and during his military service, he boxed in the ring with some hard-hitting servicemen. Randell served on the Union police force for a number of years, and he graduated with a four-year degree from the Pentecostal Bible Institute in Browerland.

One day when the Scone family had ended saying the Lord's Prayer together while holding hands, Randell turned and punched Daniel on the shoulder with a forceful, impacting punch that caught Daniel completely off guard. Daniel knew better than to try for a payback to Randell with a solid punch of his own. Daniel had come to respect Randell for his marriage to Carol, his intelligence, and his physical abilities.

Randell was demonstrating his physical prowess in some way to let Daniel know he had power in his physical strength. Randell could have been trying to shake off any Holy Spirit conviction of his sinful ways while the family held hands and said the Lord's Prayer together.

When Randell made his choice to sexually molest Marlie—whether he realized it or not—he made a choice for his and Marlie's spiritual death before the Lord. God says in Deuteronomy 30:19-20:

> I call heaven and earth as witnesses against you, that I have set before you, life and death, blessing and cursing; therefore choose life, that both you and your descendants may live; that you may love the Lord your God, that you may obey His voice, and that you may cling to Him, for He is your life and the length of your days; and that you may dwell in

the land the Lord swore to your fathers, to Abraham, Isaac, Jacob, to give them.

Death in the Biblical sense means separation from God. Only the blood of Jesus Christ can take our sins away and provide for us a way of having a new relationship with the living Lord God.

When Randell was choosing spiritual death for Marlie and himself, I was choosing life for myself with the one true God of heaven and earth, as revealed in the Holy Bible.

I had respected my brother-in-law Randell during my adolescent years, and I looked up to him with admiration as a role model. I discovered years later that Randell had been a philanderer with other women during his marriage to Carol, but I wasn't aware of all the family relationship problems until I moved along into my adult years.

My family kept many things quiet, as many families in the world do because we don't know how to deal with certain family members when they act out unusual behaviors not recognized as Christian behaviors.

Carol kept their faults from the family's attention because she was hoping that things would change for the better. She also was trying to honor the Lord by fulfilling her marriage vows before God, and she hoped to keep their marriage together by weathering the storms of life as a married couple. In many Christian families, we assume that individual family members having personal or relationship problems need to come to the end of themselves in order to allow Christ Jesus to take charge of their personal lives.

Coming to the end of themselves may take some Christians years, because many of us seem to think that we can make it in life by ourselves and we don't need the help of God and others serving as guides along the course of life's journey. Eventually Carol felt the release from the Heavenly Father to divorce her unfaithful husband and, with the passing of time, marry a good Christian man. Her marriage to Roberto Carlos is much more stable.

I came to recognize that Randell had made a crucial mistake as a Christian by getting his eyes on people, instead of keeping his eyes steadfastly on Christ Jesus. Jesus is called the Author and Finisher of our Christian faith. Many believers succumb to taking their eyes off of the One who can calm the seas of our lives and fasten their eyes on other Christians who profess Christ Jesus as Savior and Lord. When they see other Christians make critical mistakes or sin before God, they then lose faith in living the Christian faith with confidence and faith in God's Word.

Randell may have used other Christians' unfaithfulness as an excuse to pursue his own sinful course of following after the flesh by finding lonely, vulnerable, and lustful women. Randell had become another poor example of Christians who fail the Lord Jesus by loving the things that are in the world.

I recognize that Randell should have been circumspect in his Christian walk before the Lord by watching out for the following:

> Do not love the world or the things in the world. If anyone loves the world, the love of the Father is not in him. For all that is in the world—the lust of the flesh, the lust of the eyes, and the pride of life—is not of the Father but is of the world. (1 John 2:15-16 NKJV)

I discovered that Randell would find the door to repentance at times for his sinful ways only to go back to his wayward living again and again. Randell needed to learn to rely on the Lord and the help of good Christian men who could hold him accountable for his actions on a consistent basis. I recognize that there are far too many inconsistent Christians in the Christian church today.

I have discovered that walking with the Lord in purity is the sure road to holiness, which is the only way to life and power with God.

Jesus said, "Blessed are the pure in heart, For they shall see God" (Matt. 5:8 NKJV).

I wish my brother-in-law Randell could have laid hold of eternal life and the righteous principles of Jesus Christ as tenaciously as a pit bull laying hold of a dog bone with its powerful jaws. A lot of Christians have good intentions to live out their Christian walk with Christ Jesus, but when temptations come knocking at their heart's door, they flirt with the temptations, which leads to disaster and the shipwreck of their faith in God.

The Lord's solution is spoken eloquently in Psalm 119:11, which says, "Your word I have hidden in my heart, That I might not sin against You." The way to repentance requires turning from sin and its evil ways.

Solomon in the Book of Proverbs states, "He who covers his sins will not prosper, but whoever confesses and forsakes them will have mercy" (Prov. 28:13 NKJV).

Isaiah 55:7 says, "Let the wicked forsake his way, and the unrighteous man his thoughts; Let him return to the Lord, And He will have mercy on him; And to our God, For He will abundantly pardon."

The Apostle Paul, writing to Timothy, says, "Nevertheless the solid foundation of God stands, having this seal: 'The Lord knows them that are His,' and 'Let everyone who names the name of Christ depart from iniquity'" (2 Tim. 2:19).

I have come to realize that the Christian believer who is lured into the web of carnal thinking according to the world's practices must learn to reject evil imaginations.

"But each one is tempted when he is drawn away by his own desires and enticed" (James 1:14 NKJV).

God also says, "And do not be conformed to this world, but be transformed by the renewing of your mind, that you may prove what is that good and acceptable and perfect will of God" (Rom. 12:2 NKJV).

The best way to overcome persistent sexual thoughts and temptations is to recognize:

> For though we walk in the flesh, we do not war according to the flesh. For the weapons of our warfare are not carnal but mighty in God for pulling down strongholds, casting down arguments and every high thing that exalts itself against the knowledge of God, bringing every thought into captivity to the obedience of Christ. (2 Cor. 10:3-5 NKJV)

A Christian may have a fleshly thought enter his thought arena once in a while or may be bombarded with sexual thoughts, but it is imperative to cast those thoughts down and bring any carnal thinking into obedience to Christ. We can't prevent a bird from flying over our heads, but we can prevent the bird from building a nest in our hair. Christians must learn to prevent the world's way of thinking from building a safe haven of nesting in our thought life.

Learning to exchange the fleshly thoughts of the world for the thoughts that God wants us to think on must be a priority to every believer wanting to live a successful Christian life.

The Bible says:

> Finally, brethren, whatever things are true, whatever things are noble, whatever things are just, whatever things are pure, whatever things are lovely, whatever things are of good report, if there is any virtue and if there is anything praiseworthy—meditate on these things. (Phil. 4:8 NKJV)

I remember one day when I had a good talk with our father, Benjamin, about my two older sisters', Marlie's and Carol's, relationship. Benjamin commented that he thought that by taking the kids to church, they would just change by having the Word of God applied to their lives by being in church. He wasn't recognizing that each Christian principle and all applicable teachings from the Word of God needed to be applied to their lives just as he had taken the time to apply the Word of God to his personal life. Benjamin now recognized that this neglected, necessary Bible instruction had created relationship problems for the two sisters later in life.

I recognize that there are many Christian families that assume that merely going to church will automatically change their lives into the beautiful people that God wants them to be. They assume that everything will naturally change for the better and that the Bible will become their life-changing manual for every decision they make in life. Instead, they find that the individual Christian needs to, and must learn to, apply the Word of God to whatever situation he or she may be facing or dealing with in life in order to bring about the necessary changes that he or she may be expecting, wanting, and needing to happen in his or her life.

God has only good things in mind for each of us who is willing to surrender to the Lord and His will for our lives. The Lord is checking our hearts to see what is in our heart that may be hindering and holding us back from being the kind of person that He wants to make us into. God wants to mold our individual Christian lives into vessels of honor that He can use to be a blessing to others in need.

When we allow Christ Jesus to sit on the throne of our hearts, God can then direct our relationships and our personal paths in the way that we should go. We must learn to acknowledge, surrender, and submit our lives and relationships to the Lord before He can direct our lives in the way we should go. We also must learn to apply the Word of God to the situations we may face in life and to our relationships that we make in life.

I have learned from firsthand experience that things go better with Christ Jesus being at the center of our personal lives and relationships. Christ Jesus has made the difference in my life, and I would like to see every reader enjoy the benefits of having a consistent relationship with Christ Jesus, our Lord and Savior.

I recall one day when my sister Carol and my brother-in-law Randell Wikum drove over for a visit to our family home in Clover Valley. Randell was sitting in the family's comfortable cushioned chair intently reading from a book. I walked out from the kitchen with a small juice glass with water in it. I poured the water on Randell's head as a sporting gesture for fun and quickly dashed into the bathroom down the hallway, locking the dead bolt securely in place behind me.

After Randell tried the doorknob to the bathroom, I could hear him moving around in my bedroom closet directly behind the bathroom closet. I thought that Randell was trying to get at me by coming through the closet area directly behind the bathroom wall.

When I couldn't hear any more stirring around in my bedroom closet, I snuck out of the restroom to see what my brother-in-law might have been doing in my bedroom closet. To my surprise, Randell had taken my clothes off the steel bar rod and dropped them onto the floor. I was not a happy camper, and I decided to pay Randell back with a mischievous favor of my own.

I looked in the kitchen cupboard and found a box of lime Jello mix and some ketchup. I went outside to Randell and Carol's brand-new car, parked on the Scone family side lot. I poured the dried green Jello granules and red tomato ketchup onto the windshield of the new car. (I hadn't put the Jello mix and ketchup onto the car's painted surface for good reasons.)

When I went back inside the house, Randell grabbed my hands in his large left hand while he tried to spray hair spray into my face. I was moving my head back and forth, desperately trying to dodge getting sprayed in the face with the sticky hair spray.

I was successful in preventing Randell from spraying hair spray in my face, and I also was able to pull myself free from the strong grip of Randell's big hand. I discovered that I wasn't prepared for everything that Randell might have in store for me.

Randell went outside to my car and sprayed the hair spray onto my bronze metallic, two-door Chevy Vega windows. Randell also let the air out of two tires, flattening both of them where it sat on the north side lot. When I discovered what Randell had done to my tires and the windows of my car, I definitely was not pleased, to say the least.

My feud with Randell had escalated to a head when my mother, Jessica, and sister Carol called for me to stop. I, as a teenage Christian, was unhappy with Randell's actions against my personal automobile, but I reluctantly ended my ongoing battle with my older and larger opponent.

I had learned a hard lesson in life: that certain individuals are determined not to permit you to get one up on them, and they will do their level best to defeat you at whatever situation you may share with them in life. Certain people are not willing to play fair, according to the rules of the game and commonly understood boundaries of respect in relationships and human decency. Certain people are willing to hurt you if you are not careful and on your guard, to prove that they can top whatever you did or said to them. I learned the difference between a prank payback versus someone doing something against you that is over and above an equal response, which is way over the top when it comes to payback.

One day, after I had successfully pitched my Graniteville-Clover Valley Basic Legion baseball team to an exciting victory in Graniteville, I decided to go on a camping trip with my friends up Feather Creek. I had previously talked with my friend Bradly Franklyn concerning going up the Feather Creek road to an off-the-road camping area in the woods. I was going to meet up with my friends, who were going to be waiting for me up the creek after the game. I was looking forward to making the trip on my Kawasaki motorcycle to spend the night in the great outdoors. I drove home after my team's win in my mother's light green, celery-colored Rambler to load up my backpack with everything that I thought I might need for our outdoor one-day vacation.

I put my sleeping bag on the handlebars of my Kawasaki 100 motorcycle, as Jim Bronson would have in the television program *Then Came Bronson*. Then I put on my backpack with my camping necessities. I made certain that I had a good working flashlight with me before making the long trip to the campsite. As I managed to successfully ride my Kawasaki motorcycle up the Feather Creek asphalt-paved road, my headlight suddenly went out on my bike. Even with my burned-out headlight, I was determined to continue the long journey on my two-wheeled vehicle with the aid of my trusty flashlight.

Since my Kawasaki motorcycle was a clutch-operated, five-speed, heavy bike, I found that I would have to rely on holding the flashlight with my left hand as I powered the throttle handle with my right hand.

I made steady headway until I left the paved road onto the gravel section of the windy Feather Creek road. I then discovered that this method of accelerating my motorcycle while riding slowly, steadily, but ever so cautiously, on the loose shifting gravel was not met with swift progress as on the paved portion of the roadway.

I tried putting the flashlight into my mouth to light my course in the dark sections of continuous small stones and pebbles on the roadway. I also found that I was able to accelerate the throttle of my motorcycle with my right hand while I shone my flashlight with my left hand onto the side of the gravel road to maintain my position more in the center of the roadway to avoid running off the road or having a collision with the ditch or barbed wire fence. I found that my jaws got tired holding the flashlight in my mouth as another way to light my pathway through the darkened night.

I discovered that it was in my best interest to stop my bike riding periodically to give myself—and my jaws—a good break from holding my flashlight in my mouth.

Although it was a long journey and an enduring motorcycle ordeal riding through the night, I made it all the way to the dirt turnoff that would lead me to the location where my friends were camping. The good Lord was with me as I rode on into the night on the dirt trail in hopes to eventually meet up with my friends enjoying their campout.

I came to the place on the dirt road where there was a metal fence that needed to be opened in order to continue my journey to the campsite. This was an unclear point in my mind that I wasn't positive about. There hadn't been good communication before my ball game as to my friends' exact camping location. Since I couldn't see any signs of my friends along the way, I didn't realize that I needed to go through the fenced area and over a small hill section of the dirt road trail to successfully reach the area where my friends were.

Unfortunately for me, I wasn't aware that my friends were camping out just beyond the fence junction area. When I stopped my bike to call out to my friends, who might be within the sound of my voice, I never heard any response from them in the stillness of the night interrupted only by the sounds of the nearby Feather Creek.

It was a spooky situation for me, with Feather Creek making its rushing, flowing-water noise over the rocks as I steadily passed its banks leading through the mountain region. The large, looming trees and the surrounding darkness gave me a fearful foreboding; I didn't feel like hanging around there any longer. I got back on my motorcycle and rode back to a pull-off area close to Feather Creek and the dirt trail to possibly camp out by myself on a picnic table for the night.

As I rode up to the wooded picnic area in the dark night, I shone my flashlight on what appeared to be a large-eyed creature sitting stationary on top of the picnic-table bench. I became frightened when the creature didn't move one inch when I aimed the flashlight at the huge two-eyed animal. Its large eyes seemed to shine brightly back at me, never moving toward my position nor quickly darting into the woods to escape from the presence of the large boy sitting on top of my motorcycle with my helmet on.

As I held my flashlight steady at the double-eyed creature, I suddenly realized that the seemingly wild animal unwilling to budge from the picnic table was two pop cans seated close together. I decided to leave the potential campout area because of my personal encounter with a seemingly frightful creature unafraid of a showdown with a teenage boy; the spooky situation had heightened my imagination to the fears of the unknown in the great outdoors.

I rode back down to Buck State Park to hold up there for the night. I had camped out with some friends at the park before, and now that I was getting tired, I thought that possibly now was a good time to get some sleep under a covered shelter. When I turned off my motorcycle, I could hear an animal barking in the night air. I didn't know if I might meet up with a coyote or a wolf that could be in the area. I called out for the wild animal to get out of there; the fact I could not see the creature that was making the noise had brought a fear of the unknown and unseen in the dark night.

Suddenly, I heard a voice call out for me to get out of there. I wasn't about to stay there for the night and possibly have to face the people who told me to leave the park because I became frightened by the barking of what I thought might be a wild animal.

I rode my bike back out to the gravel road, and I headed for my home in Clover Valley. I eventually made it back home early in the morning when it was still dark out, and I know that the good Lord had been with me during my challenging adventure in the great outdoors.

I remember another time that God protected me and my companion from serious harm when I was riding my Kawasaki 100 motorcycle with my friend Ernest on the gravel Feather Creek road. I had been showing my friend just how good a bike rider I really was by continuously speeding up whenever I had a section of the road in which I could accelerate my vehicle and taking the turns with precision handling. I was doing a good job up to a certain point, when I saw that I needed to slow down in order to make a turn, but I realized that I was going too fast for the road conditions. My motorcycle began to slide in the gravel as I applied my front and rear brakes. As we fishtailed in the loose gravel on the heavy bike, we found ourselves heading toward the opposite shoulder of the road, nearing the edge.

I was successful in bringing my Kawasaki motorcycle to a stop, but to my regrettable surprise, Ernest had burned his bare leg on the hot tailpipe. I was truly sorry that my friend got hurt that unfortunate day, but I recognize that the situation could have been much worse had we fallen over the edge of the road on my heavy metal motorbike. I realize that I was not acting as a wise teenager with a passenger aboard, and certainly not being conservative practicing safety on a precarious gravel road.

Baseball had become a sport on which I placed a high premium in my teenage life. I believed by faith that the Lord had healed my pitching arm, which I had hurt when I was twelve years of age.

I had Pastor Neal Adams pray for my arm to be healed from the injury I experienced when I threw it out during a baseball tournament. I accepted that my arm had been healed by the Lord when Pastor Adams prayed for it to be healed. I had been chosen to be on the fifteen-year-old all-star team as a pitcher.

My teammates and I had the golden opportunity to fly up to Anchorage, Alaska, to play in a baseball tournament. While I was in Anchorage, I discovered that Tom Seaver had pitched in a similar tournament when he was fifteen years old.

I was extremely disappointed when I wasn't chosen to start the first game, and I cried tears of disappointment over what I perceived as a failed promise by one of the coaches. I was called on to start the second game, but to my chagrin, I had a poor pitching performance, which resulted in my all-star team suffering a major loss.

I heard sometime later that another pitcher on our team had said that the team would have won the tournament if he had pitched that important game. I would like to tell all of my all-star players who may have similar sentiments that I am sincerely sorry that my pitching performance resulted in my team's loss. I only wish that the other pitcher, Marvin Barnes, could have pitched the game in my place, and that he would have decisively won the game for all of his teammates.

I discovered that ping-pong was a great game to play competitively as an intense, healthy, active sport. When I was in Anchorage, Alaska, for the fifteen-year-old all-star baseball tournament, my roommate and I went over to a home where some of my other team players were staying. I found that there were some people there playing table tennis; I hadn't played the game before.

When I flew back home after the baseball tournament, I introduced the game of table tennis to my friend Dale Andrews, who was willing to go to the Clover Valley Assembly of God Church, where they had a ping-pong table in the basement.

Since baseball season was now over, I discovered that I really enjoyed playing table tennis with Dale after school as often as we could play. I started to develop into a pretty good amateur ping-pong player, who had a quick backhand and was able to keep a consistent volley of play going against some good competitive players.

I have liked healthy competition in sports as a participant and as a spectator. I have discovered that table tennis is a great game to work up a good sweat and wherein I could consistently improve my level of play with a lot of practice.

I remember playing table tennis against Pastor Neal Adams of the Clover Valley Assembly of God. Pastor Adams would hold the ping-pong paddle between his index and middle fingers, and by doing so, he could apply some really good English spins of the ping-pong ball, which I at first was not able to counter to keep the ball on the table.

When Pastor Adams would serve up a ball with some really good spin on it, I found that the ball would veer off of my paddle away from the table onto the floor. Pastor Adams consistently gave me a good cleaning in table tennis, but I was determined to practice at ping-pong until I found that I was able to defeat Pastor Adams.

I kept practicing at positioning my table-tennis paddle in ways that I found I was able to keep the ball in play. After a lot of continuous practice at table tennis, I discovered that I not only could compete against some really good talented players, but I found that I was able to win most of the games that I competed in. I have played plenty of table tennis over the years, and I still enjoy a good game of ping-pong whenever I find time to play.

I remember playing table tennis as an adult against some excellent, highly skilled ping-pong players. I discovered that I was able to hold my own against some really good players who worked with me at the William County Carrier. As a shuttle operator, I am part of a team of carrier drivers who drive the route(s) as directed by management. Each operator is responsible to drive their assigned route(s) during the shift we happen to work. A work shift may be in the morning, afternoon, or evening hours. Each carrier operator has the option to pick the shift he or she would like to work according to our individual needs. As an independent contractor, you can make some really good money as a carrier operator in a given week. It all depends on how motivated you are, how much money you are satisfied with earning, and the hours you are willing to put in each day.

I remember playing against an excellent player named Millard Judson, who told me that he was once a junior champ in table tennis. I recall that Millard gave me a nice compliment by telling me that of all the competition he had faced with the carrier company, I was the best player that he had played against. I discovered that Millard was able to come from behind whenever I had the upper ping-pong hand and find a way to defeat me in table tennis every time. I determined that although Millard consistently was able to overcome any lopsided score in which I had the lead, I would continue to play against him in hopes of finding a way to defeat him.

I remember one day that I had a young man on my personnel carrier shuttle inform me that his picture was on a magazine. As I continued to drive my carrier route to Kismet Island, the man told me that he was the third-ranked table tennis player in the United States.

When I heard this exciting news, I offered to play the young man in table tennis sometime. The man was interested in playing me at a community center on Kismet Island, but the table-tennis match never took place because the passenger was busy attending Seattle Community College. I was willing to play the man in ping-pong just for the golden opportunity of playing one of the best players in the United States, who was nationally ranked in table tennis.

I found that I continued to take a strong interest in pitching. I was good at it, but I came into a period in my life in which I was experiencing a real struggle with my pitching control. Having control problems as a teenager with pitching potential was a major disappointment to my self-esteem. I had helped my baseball teams win many games over the years, which had left me feeling emotionally confident with my peers. I felt like I didn't need to be experiencing this difficult struggle with pitching control problems in my teenage years.

It is obvious that teenagers will experience struggles, challenges, and disappointments during their adolescent years. But it can become a very difficult time in a teenager's development when his disappointments become an ongoing problem. It is important for a person's mental and emotional health to overcome his disappointments, challenges, struggles, and personal setbacks in life.

I remember a time when my Clover Valley Junior Varsity High School coach Hank Sheen put the blame squarely upon my shoulders for the team's loss of an important game. The coach was positively implying that I had intentionally lost the game by throwing the wrong pitch to the batter, who happened to make the winning hit for the opposing team.

I didn't agree with the coach's evaluation since baseball is a team sport, but I can see now from the coach's perspective just how my ineffective pitching had caused the team to give the opposing team the advantage of scoring more base runs than my team had.

I thought that the coach was truly out of line regarding his hot-tempered attitude toward myself, the critical remarks, and his evaluation of how he felt that I had blown a significant game. I had been wounded by the coach's critical remarks expressed in front of the team players, and I had felt the embarrassment of losing face before my teammates.

I maintained a quiet demeanor as my coach verbalized his hot displeasure in an angry, disrespectful, and demeaning attitude toward me. It became obvious to me that Coach Sheen needed someone to blame for the team's defeat and happened to pick me. There are some coaches who take the game so personally that during their short periods of emotional ventilation, they lose touch with the more sensitive players on the team.

As a consequence of Coach Sheen's critically excessive remarks that he vehemently spoke directly toward me after losing an important ball game, I didn't maintain any positive respect for my Clover Valley Junior Varsity High School coach for the rest of the baseball season. I continued to pitch to the best of my God-given abilities for the team, however. I lettered in my eleventh and twelfth high school years. I was successfully able to help my Clover Valley High School baseball team win at least three victories in my senior year, and the team did go on to win the state championship in the seventies. My Clover Valley Lions' baseball team was loaded with talented ballplayers, and I discovered later that the team also won the state championship the following year.

I wasn't satisfied with my pitching performance during my junior and senior years, and I decided against pursuing a college scholarship in sports after completing my senior year.

I remember that my Clover Valley Lions' High School varsity baseball coach had communicated to me that he could get me a college baseball scholarship, but at the time, I didn't have the heart that I once had for the great game of baseball to follow through with more pitching struggles. I felt that I needed to take some time postgraduation to decide what direction my life should take.

God had good things in store for me, and I needed to find the open doors that the Lord had in mind for me. I discovered that there are wonderful things in life outside of sports.

I recall a time that my Graniteville-Clover Valley Basic Legion baseball coach Bob Benson shared an interesting event with the players during one of our baseball practices. Bob Benson had played for the legendary great legion baseball coach Tom Redmond when he was only thirteen years of age. Tom Redmond coached many great-quality baseball players as the head coach of the Graniteville-Clover Valley A Legion baseball team for years.

Bob shared with the team players that he had gone back to Montana state for a baseball tournament. He went on to explain that he remembers watching an eighteen-year-old pitching to a batting cage and how his pitches were missing the screened cage used for batting practice. He told us the eighteen-year-old kid was Sandy Colfax, who was having control problems when he played legion ball. Sandy Colfax went on to be one of the legendary great baseball pitchers of all time once he was able to solve his pitching control difficulties.

This story clearly provides evidence that if a person is willing to persevere through the trials of hard, adverse, and difficult times, he can look forward to bigger, better, and greater things in his pursuit for the good things in life and possibly see his life's dreams fulfilled.

I remember getting the call from Coach Bob, and I discovered that I would pitch against Gary Holland, a tall, hard-throwing, fastball hurler from Carltonville, who had excellent pitching skills, with good control. I remember Gary having a long, full head of hair that stuck out from the sides and back of his ball cap. I would pitch for the Graniteville-Clover Valley Basic Legion baseball team against Gary, representing a fundamentally sound team appropriately named the Carltonville Bulldogs, because they were stubborn about giving up any runs at the Liberty City Park.

Gary was throwing consistent high heat against the Graniteville-Clover Valley Basic Legion team when it became my turn to bat. I stepped up to the plate, only to go down on three straight fastballs from Gary, looking like aspirin tablets sailing right across the plate into the catcher's glove. I looked like a blind man looking for a black cat in a dark room. My hitting abilities were simply no match against the superior pitching opposition, and Gary wasn't giving up any free passes on base by walking a batter from four balls out of the strike zone surrendering a walk.

My teammates put up a hearty hitting scrimmage against Gary, with a number of strikeouts, but we couldn't put together a string of hits to produce any runs against the directly over-the-top, hard-throwing, right-handed pitcher who handsomely defeated the Graniteville-Clover Valley Basic Legion baseball team five to nothing that day. Unfortunately, I found along with my teammates that we were simply not fierce competition against the future major league pitcher. I discovered years after my pitching debut against Gary Holland that he was drafted by the California Angels.

During the game, I had one of my teammates, Darrin Redmond, give me a verbal reprimand for the lack of faith I had demonstrated as my team was not making any scoring progress against Gary Holland. I knew that Darrin was telling me the truth about the comments I had made during the game and my attitude, which revealed my discouragement in the face of our lack of hitting success against Gary.

I was surprised by Darrin's truthful evaluation of my lack of possessing any winning psychology, which had clearly diminished against such a fierce pitching opponent as Gary.

The Graniteville-Clover Valley Basic Legion team still lost the game, but it was a good lesson for me to remember that no matter what the game, situation, or score standings might be, it is always important to maintain a winning psychological attitude that your team can make a comeback to win the game in the end.

With God, all things are possible to them who believe, and hopefully your team will have a better outing next time you face the same pitcher provided you have put in a lot of practice on the things that your team may be weak in.

I discovered years later that Gary went on to pitch professionally in the major leagues, with a ninety-five-mile-an-hour fastball. Gary continued pitching professionally in the major leagues as a naturally gifted, all-around talented athlete until he walked away from pitching in the major leagues one day. I think it was pretty neat that I had the opportunity to pitch against a future major league pitcher.

I recall the tremendous influence that Dwayne Friend had on my Christian witnessing for Christ Jesus. I remember how one of my classmates, Glen Sims, crumpled up a gospel tract that I handed to him and threw it on the floor as a demonstration of defiance against my Christian witnessing. Glen did pick it up as if he were merely kidding, but it was probably an outward manifestation of an attitude of disgust for my consistent sharing of my faith with others whenever I had an open door to witness. Dwayne Friend was a bold, powerful, lay-it-on-the-line-and-tell-it-like-it-is evangelist for Jesus Christ.

I desired to witness for my Lord and Savior Jesus Christ in hopes of leading lost souls to the Lord, so I also became willing to reach out to others for Jesus as Dwayne was doing by sharing my faith with people. I found an effective method of reaching others for Christ was by handing out gospel tracts. The good news of how someone could be saved from their sins, invite Jesus into their hearts, and have eternal life by believing on the Lamb of God, Jesus Christ, was clearly communicated in each gospel tract I would hand to a prospect for Christ.

I found I wasn't intimidated by the act of rejection of the good news of salvation as clearly explained in the gospel tract. One day Brad Allen, a classmate of mine, mentioned to me as I handed him a gospel tract titled "Holy Joe," "You're just like him," implying that I was similar in the type of a witness for Jesus Christ as Holy Joe was in the gospel tract I had handed to Brad. I accepted the title as a compliment of my consistent living of a righteous and godly Christian life and as a witness for Christ, of which the world needs to see more. I recognize that there are far too many inconsistent Christians in the Christian church today.

I liked to imitate and memorize certain things that Dwayne Friend would say in his evangelistic crusades. Dwayne was an effective communicator for Christ Jesus during his soul-saving meetings, wherein he used catchy phrases and sayings to capture the attention of the audience.

Dwayne said, "The man who testifies for God by the yard, but lives for him by the inch, ought to be kicked by the foot."

I remember Dwayne saying, "If talking were effective, there are scores and scores of men who would move a mountain off its base and move it back again. But as a language stated true and blunt, they're never worth a dime to lift 'cause all they do is grunt."

Dwayne also said, "Some Christians' faces are so long they look like a Missouri mule," referring to believers in Christ Jesus who don't manifest the joy of the Lord on their faces but choose to reveal a more sour and sullen Christian appearance as a gloomy witness for the Lord.

Dwayne would say, "Their tongues are so long you could roll a biscuit on it."

When he referred to how high his brother Harold could sing, he said, "He sings higher than a hawk's nest."

I remember a powerful saying Dwayne Friend used in a sermon on soul winning. He said, "Do you know that God can't use you until you admit that you're not worth a dime? When you finally admit it, God can use your life." I have remembered that great truth in my own personal life in wanting to be a witness for the Lord and in my approach with God throughout the years.

I remember Dwayne sharing about a man named Jim, who had heard some singing coming from a church on a cold winter night. Jim left the church that night after listening to the singing, only to return the next business day.

The pastor was in his study room when he observed Jim walk down the aisle to kneel in prayer at the altar. The pastor heard Jim say while kneeling, "Jesus, this is Jim." That's all Jim said. He then got up and walked out of the church.

Dwayne shared that Jim got hit by a truck while he was walking out, and his body sailed through the air and landed against some rocks. Jim was taken to the hospital in bad shape. The pastor of the church where

Jim had knelt in prayer heard that he was in the hospital, and he went in to see him.

As the pastor stood near Jim, he heard a voice say, "Jim, this is Jesus. I've come to heal you."

Dwayne shared that Jesus had healed Jim and Jim had gone into the ministry. I was really touched spiritually and emotionally by this wonderful story about a man named Jim.

The next Wednesday night, I decided to share the amazing story about Jim, whom Jesus had healed, and how he had gone into the ministry with the small congregation at the Clover Valley Assembly of God Church.

As I took my turn to share the incredible story with the people in attendance that night, I began to get emotionally broken up, and I began to cry. The blessed Holy Spirit was working in my heart and life as a teenager, and I was having a difficult time telling this emotionally moving story to the people.

God was using the story of the man named Jim as told by Dwayne Friend to do something special spiritually and emotionally in my young Christian life. God is so good, kind, and loving to those who love Him and the people who are willing to place their faith in Him and His finished work on the cross of Calvary.

I remember one night when I drove out of state to Graniteville, to attend a Tabernacle Church service. They had a guest speaker who shared how God had helped him and the men who were in his special frogmen military operation during a time of war against German soldiers occupying a concrete fortress. The man of God shared a fascinating story in detail of how God had protected him during this special operation, which caught the occupying German soldiers by surprise.

After the special speaker had shared his incredible story in chronological order of the events that had taken place in the dark of night, I reflected on how this man of God was truly a man of tremendous prayer with power. I thought how great it would be to be an effective man of God like this man was. It was obvious that this man knew how to get results through his prayers on behalf of their military operation, which had been carried out with great success. I was impressed to hear the wonderful story of how God had protected this precious man of God and his men during a time of war.

I recall another night that I drove out of state to Graniteville to attend the Tabernacle Church again. This time the pastor of the church did something unusual, which took me by surprise. I remember how Pastor Cliff Flores pointed me out in the church to come forward to the front of the church as the congregation looked on.

I can remember that when I stepped out into the aisle of the church, I felt the presence of the Lord meet me there before I walked forward. Once I stepped out in obedience to the calling of the man of God, the Spirit of the Lord met me in the aisle. It was surprising to me to immediately feel God's presence suddenly meet me there as I continued to walk forward to the front of the church.

Before I stepped out in obedience to the call of God, the pastor of the church could spiritually visualize the calling on my life. God was preparing me for the work of the ministry in whatever direction that would take. I remember that there were kids at school who would tell me that I was going to be a preacher.

When I shared my faith with my friends and others, I was doing the work of the ministry even if I wasn't officially preaching, teaching, or ministering behind a pulpit in front of a church congregation.

I recall going on a hunting trip with my good friend Jay LeBlanc. Jay had purchased a doe tag, and he invited me to go deer hunting with him. We drove from Clover Valley, up the Sussan River to hunt the surrounding hills in the Grand River area. Jay and I hiked over a number of hills that Saturday, only to come up empty of seeing any deer, let alone bringing down a good-sized doe.

Since Jay had a good hunting rifle with a scope, I was leaving all the shooting for him to bag himself a qualified deer having the right size and weight that would meet the standards of the fish and game department. When Jay decided to give up hunting for the day, we headed back down the Grand River road, keeping an eye out for any deer sightings along the way.

Suddenly I spotted what I thought for sure was a mountain lion on the side of the hill across from the Grand River. As the two teenagers traveled closer to the area where the big cat was sighted roaming the hillside, Jay recognized that the large-tailed animal wasn't a mountain lion at all. The long-tailed, four-footed creature turned out to be a woolly sheep with a big tail that hadn't been cut off by its owner.

Jay began laughing at me for my mistaken animal identification; it wasn't a large-tailed, furry animal roaming the hills for prey as a big puma cat would, but a woolly-tailed sheep roaming the hills for nourishing grass to consume.

I wasn't a hunter experienced at distinguishing the species of large game to hunt, nor was I an Eagle Scout able to spot big game for Jay when he needed me to. Jay recognized my inexperience at hunting, and he had himself a good laugh over the inaccurate sighting.

—⁓⦾⦿⦾⁓—

After Marlie had her second child, named Garth, she asked me if I would babysit him one day because she had things to do. I was willing to watch over Garth as his uncle and take care of the new addition to the family. After watching over Garth for a while, I discovered that it was time to change his diaper. I laid Garth down on a newspaper for the necessary change. I wasn't the most experienced diaper changer in the world, but I was willing to do my best at making things more comfortable for my baby nephew. I successfully made the diaper change to the best of my hands inexperienced at handling safety pins, and I thought that Garth was good to go now for happier times in the Scone family home.

When Garth was back with his mother, it was Marlie's turn to change his diaper. She later told me that she could read the newspaper print imprinted on his butt. Marlie admitted to me that she could only clearly read the word "the" and everything else was a blur. It must have made for some interesting reading. Marlie, as a young mother had me babysit, and without my knowing that laying Garth down on a Graniteville newspaper to make the necessary diaper change would result in leaving behind some incriminating evidence of precisely what my method was of changing my nephew's wet. absorbent cloth diaper, adding a sensitive sense of tender care and humor by providing newspaper print to his baby bottom. I have come to realize that many things do turn out for good in the end in more ways than one.

When Garth was a young child, Marlie brought him over to the Scone family home because she had things to take care of again. Garth was a cute little boy, who would have baby boo-boos now and then. That particular day, Garth happened to have himself a hard, painful fall onto the linoleum floor in the living room. Rather than focusing my attention on Garth's infantile injury, which could have caused him to cry even more, I focused my attention on the floor being possibly damaged from the fall to deflect

Garth's focus away from his pain. I walked over to the area he had fallen onto, and I got down to examine the floor as if I were making sure that the floor wasn't indented from Garth's big fall.

When Garth saw me paying attention to see if the floor was all right, he suddenly stopped crying and made his own surface inspection of the linoleum flooring. After Garth had made a thorough examination to be sure the floor wasn't damaged from his great fall, he found that life was now prepared for more of little Garth to enjoy bigger things and better times through his experiences of exploring new discoveries in the Scone family home.

When Marlie had her third child, she named him Travis. He provided a lot of humorous times for their household. Travis liked to watch *Tarzan* on television, and one day he made an interesting comment to Marlie that caused her to laugh. Travis had watched enough of the Tarzan movies for him to conclude that something was missing from his jungle life and activities. He wondered aloud why Tarzan never went to the bathroom. Had I been there when young Travis made his humorous observation, I might have shared with my young nephew that Tarzan probably knew how to hold it. Travis might not have understood the witty comeback provided by his uncle, but it could have brought forth a humorous response from the others watching.

Travis heard one Sunday from their Christian church that Jesus lives big in your heart and life. When he saw a 350-pound woman who attended their church, named Shelley Moore, he said to her, "Shelley, I know why you're so big. It's because Jesus lives big in your heart and life." He stretched out his arms real wide.

I enjoyed playing with Garth and Travis over the years as they were growing up. I had a good time playing baseball, tennis, and board games like *Monopoly*, and taking them out for some good-tasting fast food at McDonald's or to the Arctic Circle for a tasty hamburger, French fries, and an ice-cold drink, or if they preferred, a milkshake.

My two young nephews and niece and I always took time to thank the Lord for the good food He provided for us to eat.

I recall one Sunday afternoon when I had a negative encounter with my father, Benjamin. I was seated on the side of the dinner table, and my mother, Jessica, and my dad were seated opposite at the head of the table.

I don't recall what I said at the time, but I remember making a negative remark about my dad in front of him. I had picked up on a critical spirit that Jessica had toward Benjamin, and now I had expressed that same critical spirit toward my father. Benjamin stood up, and he wanted to discipline me for my critical attitude.

I wasn't aware of it at the time, but I had dishonored my father by the negative comment that I had made about him. Benjamin tried to hold both of my hands, and he tried to slap me in the face in the kitchen.

I was now a strong seventeen-year-old athlete who had lifted weights growing up, and I shoved my father away from me in anger and told him to leave me alone. Benjamin recognized the power in my shove, and he proceeded to back down from trying to discipline his son over what I had said to him in a critical tone of voice. I left the kitchen and went to my room, where I had a good cry over what had just taken place with my dad.

I had a rude awakening that my father didn't appreciate my negative faultfinding attitude. I later apologized for what I had said to my dad that Sunday afternoon.

The next day when I came home from school, I inquired of my mother, Jessica, why she was bucking dad all the time. By now, I had done a lot of thinking about Sunday's negative encounter with my father, and I was looking for an answer why I might be picking up on a critical spirit from her about my dad. I was still a young Christian, and I needed to do some more growing up spiritually in my relationship toward my father.

Jessica related to me that there was a time that she had seen the next-door neighbor mistreat his little woman, and she found herself determining that she wasn't going to submit herself to any man in her life. Mother had decided to take that stand when she was only nine years old, and it was manifesting itself through having a critical spirit now as a married woman. I didn't understand everything that Jessica was telling me after the Sunday incident with my dad, but I had awakened to the fact that my attitude toward my father needed to change for the better for the Lord's sake.

I came to the realization that I needed to have the right attitude toward my dad, and the Lord helped me to see that I needed to have a God-honoring relationship with Him and my father. Benjamin and I seemed to relate better as I grew in my understanding of the ways of the Lord.

Thank the Lord, I never had another bad attitude toward my dad after that day.

I attended a Future Living class when I was going to Clover Valley High School in my senior year. My teacher, Judith Dempsy, wanted to show the class a film of a woman giving birth. As I was watching the woman giving birth in the film, I became queasy at the sight of blood and began to feel light-headed. I found myself putting my head down in the back of the class because I felt like I was going to faint. I never did like the sight of blood—especially my own.

I recall a time when I was in junior high school when I began to feel faint during my physical education class as I watched a man having his chest cut open because of cancer. When I saw the blood and the black cancer cells inside of the man's chest, I put my head down as I sensed I was getting light-headed and feeling like I was going to faint. I had a sensitive nature about me when it came to the sight of blood that other people do not seem to have a problem with.

I reflect back to an earlier time while attending Jefferson Middle High School in Clover Valley. I had successfully cut out a pen holder using the jigsaw blade as assigned by the wood shop teacher, Benny Rogers. One of my classmates, Tim Dickson, wasn't as confident about using the jigsaw machine. I was willing to help out a fellow classmate, and I began to push the wooden board toward the thin saw blade with my left thumb.

I wasn't paying attention to how close my thumb was to the blade when I suddenly felt the jigsaw blade cutting into the tip of my thumb. I quickly pulled my hand away and tightly wrapped my fingers around my thumb. When I saw the blood on my hand from the cut, I began moving quickly over to my workbench to sit down on the floor.

When my teacher, Mr. Rogers, saw me leaning back against the workbench and sitting on the floor feeling faint concerning my cut, bloody thumb, he thought it was hilarious. I wasn't amused by Mr. Roger's lighthearted attitude toward my thumb's encounter with the thin saw blade that had caught me by surprise.

I am grateful that the tip of my thumb wasn't cut off at the time of the incident. I still carry a thin cut mark as evidence of my distracted carelessness on the tip of my thumb to this day as a result of my encounter with the jigsaw blade in my woodshop class.

I realize I didn't jig fast enough when the jig was up.

THE ADULT YEARS

After I graduated from Clover Valley High School, I applied for summer work at Bridge Port City Foods. I was hired on as a combine operator working in the pea harvest for the sum of $3.25 an hour. My coworkers and I would drive combines to harvest peas in large fields on a twelve-hour shift from sundown to sunrise.

I remember coming home one morning after riding my combine, which had automatic levelers, to take a bath. The automatic levelers help the combines to adjust to going up and down hills and when a combine operator was harvesting peas on the sides of the hills.

After pouring my bathwater, I sat down to enjoy a good bath to clean off all the dirt that had accumulated on me from driving the combine in the dusty pea fields. When I sat down in the bathtub, it seemed like it was beginning to move around me. It took a short while for my mind and body to adjust to me sitting in the bathtub, realizing that I was no longer riding my combine at work.

I found that the motion I experienced from driving the combine all night, I was now feeling in my mind since it had been recorded on my memory bank.

I remember one night it was extremely cold. When I took my lunch break, I hovered close to the large combine engine, which helped to keep me warm during the unusually chilly night. That rare night during the summer months felt more like a cold winter night to me.

I was assigned to drive a swather for the pea harvest one summer. Driving the swather was a lot faster than a combine harvesting the peas, and if one was good at swathing, he could take a rest as the combines kept operating at a much slower pace.

Once the pea harvest came to an end, my two friends Brett Roberts and Shawn Anderson and I decided to go on an oceanic fishing trip. Brett had been on the Pacific Ocean on a number of occasions, whereas Shawn and I had not. We rented an eighteen-foot runabout and headed out of the inlet of Lapush, Washington, to the wide open sea to land a big king or silver salmon. Shawn had driven a boat on the Sussan River and also on some lakes before.

Brett asked one skipper of a charter boat how things were on the ocean that day, and the skipper responded that there were kicker boats coming in but he thought it was all right to go out. Brett had more knowledge of oceanic experiences so he was the skipper, and Shawn became the driver of our fast-running seaworthy vessel.

Shawn seemed confident as he was running the boat in the inlet, but when we were ready to leave the harbor and enter the blue ocean waters, there was a large wave coming directly at us.

Shawn saw the big wave coming at us and said, "Oh, jazz."

Our boat went up into the air with our collision with the huge wave, and Shawn immediately pulled back on the engine throttle to slow our speed. Wave after wave kept coming at us and pushing our boat back toward the rocks behind us. Brett called out to Shawn to give it more throttle to move us away from being shipwrecked on the rocks. Shawn gave the boat more throttle thrust to move us out into the house-sized waves, and we were on our way out to sea.

Brett, Shawn, and I went out on the mighty Pacific Ocean in what Brett later described as the worst weather he'd ever experienced. The large waves were capping, and the three friends went up with one wave and were able to see a large cargo ship off in a distance; when we went down with a huge wave, we could see nothing but sky and large surrounding waves. This was my first time being on the high seas, and I found myself vomiting from all the rocking and rolling with the swelling waves.

The three amigos were determined to catch some salmon, and we kept at it until I happened to catch a salmon only to have it bite the line and disappear into the vast waters.

After fishing for some time, my friends and I decided to call it quits for a while and head back in for a break from dealing with the powerful ocean waves.

When back on land, I had a drink of water and a chocolate candy bar that seemed to hit the spot. I no longer had a queasy stomach from the rolling waves; rather, I discovered that I was now willing to go out fishing again. After approximately an hour of break time on land, we were all ready to go back out on the mounting ocean waters again to do some more fishing.

I recall a wooden plaque that my father, Benjamin, had in the basement. The "Anglers Prayer" read as follows:

"Lord, Give Me a Fish So Big That Even I, in Telling of It Afterward, May Never Need to Lie . . ."

Brett, Shawn, and I were hoping to catch a number of good-sized salmon we would be proud to show the family and that would make for some good eating later around the dinner table.

I remember my dad sharing with me about a time when he had gone fishing with Jessica, Randell Wikum, and Carol. The four had gone on a campout that included some fishing. Benjamin caught himself a large rainbow trout that he was quite proud of. He brought it back to their campsite and placed the big fish into a pail of water to keep it fresh. He then proceeded to go into the tent to take a nap, which he always liked to do after his fishing labors.

Later, when he went to look for his fourteen-inch trout, it was nowhere to be found. When he questioned Randell about it, he just patted his stomach and told Benjamin that it had made for some good eating.

Needless to say, my father was not pleased with his son-in-law, Randell Wikum, that day. Benjamin was planning on bringing the large rainbow trout home to show off his successful fishing outing to family, neighbors, and friends, but he found that he wasn't going to get the chance to show off his prize fish to anybody thanks to Randell.

I liked to let my fishing line out a long distance behind the fishing boat. I wasn't an experienced salmon fisherman, but I was up for being a good sport about reeling in a large fish that would make for some good eating later.

I caught another salmon on my hook, and this time Brett, who was a much more experienced fisherman, took control of my pole to ensure that this salmon would not get away. When the salmon was to the back of the boat, Shawn reached down to catch the large fish in his net.

It turned out that I caught the only silver salmon for the day. After fishing for what seemed like a good while, I threw up again. As before, I put my head down as Shawn navigated the eighteen-foot runabout back toward land for the final time. As we began heading back, Shawn was driving rather quickly, doing a good job of staying out in front of a good-sized wave directly behind the boat.

When Shawn turned the seaworthy vessel sideways to make his turn into the harbor, a large wave almost capsized the boat. God was with us that day as we proceeded to make the long trip back home. My friends shared the near misfortune with me after we were back on land again.

On the way back to Clover Valley, we dropped off Shawn in Refus, where he lived with his wife, Mary Jo.

In the fall I applied for employment at the Crest Forest Industries, which is now Timberland Forest Industries. I found that I didn't have to wait long before I received a phone call to come in for an interview.

I later was contacted by phone to come to work at the sawmill plant located in east Graniteville. I found that I didn't care for the tough work conditions at the sawmill, and I decided to quit after only a few months' employment.

After working at the mill, I was able to work with my friend Brett for a short time putting cedar shakes on people's roofs. It was beginning to get colder in Clover Valley, and I didn't continue to work with Brett putting cedar shakes on people's homes.

I found that I was out of work for the rest of the year, but since I was still living at home with my parents, I wasn't too concerned about being without employment.

The following year I was able to reapply at the Crest Forest Industries sawmill plant. I was grateful that I was given another opportunity to work at the CFI sawmill. I discovered that it's better being employed making money working hard than being unemployed and broke.

I found that I was making good money at the sawmill, and I was able to purchase my first car with the money I was earning. I found that I could make large payments toward my new bronze metallic, two-door Chevy Vega. I chose the car for its sporty look, and I liked having a clutch four-speed vehicle to drive to work and get around town.

God was blessing me as I continued to live at home with my parents, work at the sawmill, and attend the Clover Valley Assembly of God Church.

My friend Jay LeBlanc called me one day and told me about a Christian woman who was just like me. Jay was so incredibly impressed with this special Christian lady who worked at the Clover Valley Care Center along with Jay that he just knew his coworker Olivia Knutson and I had to meet sometime.

Jay encouraged me to give Olivia a call as soon as I possibly could. Jay had checked with Olivia to see if it was all right for me to call her sometime, and she had agreed. Olivia and I had a good conversation together over the phone before we went out on our first date.

I soon discovered that I really liked Olivia's sweet personality, and I liked spending time with her. I found myself enjoying playing miniature golf which was next to the bowling alley on Cloverland Street in Clover Valley with Olivia. I also enjoyed taking Olivia to Wanpa Lake in the state of Idaho and going to her First Baptist Church in Clover Valley to see a Christian film called *The Rapture.*

I was falling in love with this pretty brunette Christian woman. As Olivia and I were getting to know one another, Olivia shared with me that she was going to attend Western Baptist College in Salem, Oregon. I found myself saddened by the news of her leaving to a separate state, but I was encouraged that she was still interested in corresponding with me via letters and phone calls.

Jay recognized that I was thinking a lot about Olivia after she had gone away to the Christian college. Olivia had also thought about me during her absence, and she invited me to come down for a nice visit. Olivia wanted me to come down to see her, and she made me think she had missed me. I discovered that Jay was willing to make the long trip with me from Clover Valley to Salem, Oregon, the state capital, south of Portland, Oregon.

After Jay and I arrived at the Baptist College, Olivia wanted me to meet with a conservative Baptist leader who was convinced that the baptism of the Holy Spirit with the evidence of speaking in other tongues was not for believers today.

I had spoken in tongues before, and I believed that the gift of tongues was for us today.

I listened carefully to what Lenny Myers had to say about his personal experience of speaking in tongues. He didn't believe it was real even though he told me that he had spoken in tongues at a Christian gathering before. Lenny didn't experience the power that comes with speaking in other tongues, as Jesus had promised to his disciples.

I disagreed with Lenny, but I didn't think it was my place at the time to try to convince him that what the Bible says about speaking in tongues—*"God says, 'For the promise is to you and to your children, and to all who are afar off, as many as the Lord our God shall call'"*—means exactly that God is willing to give to all Christian believers open to His free gift (Acts 2:38-39).

Olivia had been influenced by Baptist Christian leaders like Lenny and teachers at the Bible school she was listening to in her classes. Olivia came to the conclusion that there definitely was a major difference between her Baptist faith that speaking in tongues was not for today and what Kurtess's Pentecostal-believing Assembly of God Church believed in.

I was seeing signs in Olivia's attitude toward what I believed in and by the things she had communicated to me that things were cooling off in our relationship together.

"How can two walk together except they are in agreement?" (Amos 3:3).

Olivia, Jay, and I went on a drive together in Salem, Oregon, that revealed how Olivia honestly felt about her relationship with me. During the course of our drive in Jay's truck, Olivia kindly mentioned that Jay was cute. Olivia told Jay that she had always felt that he was handsome.

Olivia made it perfectly clear that she never felt that I was handsome, and when I heard her preferential words spoken so freely toward Jay, it was very obvious to me that she didn't really love me from the heart. As I rode along with Jay and Olivia quietly listening to the sweet talk Olivia was making toward Jay, while conspicuously neglecting any kind words toward me, I was hurt by the special treatment Olivia was giving to Jay and felt that she was being disrespectful of my love for her.

The words spoken sweetly to Jay by who I *thought* was my girlfriend who supposedly loved me were a clear indication that Olivia's heart really wasn't fixed on me. It was Olivia who had given me an open invitation to come down to Western Baptist College, but she clearly did not truly love me.

The trip to see Olivia turned out to be a painful one for me, but it helped me to see the obvious: that my relationship with Olivia was not worth pursuing. Olivia made it evident that she was willing to have me change from my doctrinal position of believing in the baptism of the Holy Spirit with the initial evidence of speaking in other tongues to possibly keep the relationship doors open with her. I decided not to break tradition with the Pentecostal belief in the power of the Holy Spirit as was experienced by the disciples of Jesus Christ in the upper room in Acts 2:4.

I came to realize that there were more fish in the sea of dating and courtship than just Olivia Knutson.

When I graduated from Clover Valley High School, my family was in the stands during the ceremony procession. I thought that it was a good ceremony, and all of my classmates at Clover Valley High School managed to successfully get through the graduation ceremony in an orderly, formal manner.

After the graduation, the Scone family had our picture taken, with me as the graduate. As usual, I was always interested in taking a close look at the graduation picture to see how I looked in the photo once my mother had the pictures developed. I especially closely examined how my nose appeared in the graduation picture and whether it appeared too large, prominent, and noticeably conspicuous.

I knew that if I noticed my nose, then others who happened to take a look at the picture would be able to observe my bulbous tip nose as well.

I did the same thing with all of my pictures growing up and also as an adult. Ever since I was in Cloverdale Elementary School, I was quick to notice what my nose looked like in each individual picture and every family photo. I wanted to especially know whether my smelling apparatus looked good in the picture with me in it.

Each time that I observed that my nose was too conspicuous to overlook in a family picture, it caused me to become self-conscious about my nose once more. I was keenly aware that my nose was larger than most noses on peoples' faces, and this made me feel insecure and more self-conscious about my physical appearance.

My sensitivity regarding my nose would be a lifelong struggle, in which I would need God's grace to sustain me throughout the years.

I recall a time when I was attending Jefferson Middle High School in Clover Valley. My science teacher, Albert Scoggins, brought colored eggs to our class. He placed them in warm incubators for them to hatch as our science experiment. Later, when the eggs hatched, I was able to bring two pink baby chicks home with me, and I found that I took an interest in raising the little chicks up from being tiny baby fowls until I was able to give them away to the Arthers, who already had chickens.

I would go out in the night to catch night crawlers to feed to my chicks. They loved to eat all the large worms that I would feed them until their chests would swell up like a balloon inside of them. My small chicks loved all the night crawlers I could find to feed them, and they loved to eat chicken feed and bugs.

I had my own Farmer-John experience raising the chicks into full-grown chickens, and I found that it was indeed an interesting and good experience at that.

One day my mother, Jessica, took a picture of me with the two baby chicks on each of my shoulders, my black dog Nubbin laying on his back on my right arm, and the family's black and white pet cat Bo laying on his back while on my left arm.

It turned out to be quite a colorful picture with me being close to my animals wearing my blue high-water pants. After the picture was developed, I was conscientiously interested in seeing what my nose looked like in the picture. Once again, I found myself emotionally discouraged when I observed that my bulbous nose stood out as the most embarrassingly noticeable physical facial feature; this caused more self-conscious sensitivity to grow inside of me. I hadn't yet progressed in my Christian faith in the finished work of the cross of Christ Jesus when I was in my eighth-grade science class, but I would continue to be sensitive about my physical features even after I became a genuine born-again Christian.

I later learned that God was using my physical characteristics to build character qualities in me that only He could create for my good. God's ways and purposes are not our ways, but He knows what it requires to produce good character in each of His children for His glory.

I remember one event working at the Crest Forest Industries sawmill in Graniteville, where I was injured on the job. I recall a painful incident when I was using a long push bar that looked like a metal rocket to push a large log that wasn't moving on the sawmill deck toward the cutoff saw.

I lifted the heavy push bar, which had a bent metal prong underneath it, into the stationary chain positioned in a steel sleeve on the deck. Once I had the push bar ready for the deck operator to move the chains, the sudden thrust of the chain below me caused the push bar to twist, and I lost control of the torpedo-shaped push bar.

I quickly reacted to catch the falling push bar, and without thinking of what I was doing, my right index finger was caught between the push bar and the steel sleeve housing the steel chain. I found myself reacting in pain, and I began moving quickly around the deck, sensing the acute pain in my finger.

My lead man, Albert Eastlund, took me over to the restroom to run some cold water over my painful cut finger. After cool water ran over my finger, Albert was going to take me down to the first aid department for them to bandage my finger.

Albert thought that I was all right after my injury, but to my surprise, right before the restroom doorway, I fainted from the traumatic experience of having cold running water flow over my injured digit and from seeing my own blood oozing from my finger.

Albert revived me from fainting and assisted me down to the first aid department. After having my finger bandaged by the caring nurse, I was ready to resume my work on the sawmill deck.

I still carry the scar on my index finger, which provides the white-shaped appearance of a fingernail attempting to grow through the skin.

I recall a time when I was working in the Crest Forest Industries sawmill that I had an unusual spiritual experience that I never had before up until then. I had come to know spiritual touches from the Lord, which I could physically feel. I knew what it was to enjoy the joy of the Lord, and what it felt like to experience a spiritual restoration in my heart and soul after going through a dry spell.

This particular day, I felt what I would later describe to a friend as a spiritual snowball or meteorite coming right through my silver-colored hard hat. I took mental note of this unusual sensation from the Lord and kept on doing my work at the sawmill. I knew what it was like to have a parakeet on my head, finger, and shoulders before, and now I was beginning to experience spiritual sensations on my head that were similar to the light parakeet-feet sensations I had felt when my parakeet Pretty Pete would land on my hair. I eventually came to the scriptural realization that the Lord as my good Shepherd was reassuring me that He was with me by laying His blessed hand upon my life, and the pouring on or painting my life with the anointing of oil, which is symbolic of the Holy Spirit coming upon an individual Christian's life for His service and ministry. A couple of verses to support my thinking on the above are: "You prepare a table before me in the presence of my enemies; You anoint my head with oil; my cup runs over" (Ps. 23:5, NKJV). "You have hedged me behind and before, And laid Your hand upon me. Such knowledge is too wonderful for me; It is high, I cannot attain it" (Ps. 139:5-6, NKJV).

That night after work, I went into the bathroom at home to stand in front of the mirror. With my work helmet off, I began to check and see if I could visibly observe any impressions on my hair of what felt like parakeet-feet impressions.

I wasn't able to see any visible impressions on my hair that day, but I knew this wasn't something I was imagining. Although I could feel the sensations on my hair, I wasn't quite sure what this could mean. When I read in Holy Scripture that God had anointed David's head with oil and how the Holy Spirit came down upon Jesus in the form of a dove, I came to the realization that these touches from the Lord were signs that God truly hadn't forgotten me. He was showing how much He loved me by providing spiritual manifestations of His loving and protective hand on my life.

I found that my father, Benjamin, and I enjoyed going hunting together. We would take Benjamin's Remington .22 rifle and his Classic Sharp Shot .20-gauge shotgun out to hopefully shoot a rabbit or bag some quail and pheasants during our outdoor hunting experience. Unfortunately our outdoor hunting activities were not the most successful hunting ventures as far as bagging any wild birds, but we liked getting out of town for the hunting experience anyway.

I found that my relationship with my father improved as I grew older, and especially as I grew spiritually in my understanding of the ways of the Lord as an adult. My father and I would have long talks together discussing the good things of God, end-time events we could see shaping up in what many Christians believe are the last days, and how the Lord is at work in Christian lives today.

We also found that our long discussions could include some good, hearty, humorous times in which we would begin laughing together over seemingly little things that would hit our funny bones with our good sense of humor.

Benjamin and I bonded together spiritually through going hunting or fishing together and through sharing laughter with one another over things that we considered humorous as father and son.

I remember a haircut experience when my father, Benjamin, was cutting my hair in our basement. Benjamin had a barber chair that he had transported to our home and placed in the basement for him to cut hair at home. I wanted my father to cut my hair just right, because I had fine hair and I was especially sensitive about how my haircut looked on me.

After Benjamin thought he had done a good job cutting my hair, I went upstairs to inspect my haircut in front of the bathroom mirror. I thought that my haircut needed to be evenly balanced, so I came back downstairs to have Benjamin try to make some precise changes.

After each correction, I would inspect my father's work in the bathroom mirror. Finally, when my finicky attitude about y hair was causing Benjamin to grow weary with the length of the haircut experience, he said, "When I get through, it's going to be a $50 haircut."

I thought that comment was pretty good coming from my dad, but my father caught me by complete surprise with an unexpected remark when he said to me, "That's where the side of your head is caved in." Benjamin and I began to have ourselves a good long laugh about his comment. The moment struck a funny chord that brought total laughter in agreement that we both could relate to.

One day I was having a good talk with Isaac Nelson, who was attending Union Theology Institute. I appreciated talking to Isaac and learning about what I could expect should I decide to go to the Union Theology Institute.

At a later time, I had a separate talk with Hal Matheson, who also was attending Union Theology Institute. The more I thought about attending the Theology Institute, the more I began to see the importance of going to a Christian school that had excellent Bible teachers with an emphasis strictly on the Word of God to learn more about the things of God.

I couldn't see myself being a lifer at the Crest Forest Industries sawmill although I was making good money at the time.

I took the next step by contacting the Bible school to find out if I could start attending the Christian school. I talked to the Theology Institute's registrar, Pastor Peter Sampson, who was good about getting me enrolled for the fall semester.

In the fall, I began attending Union Theology Institute in Union. I found that I enjoyed attending the Institute, and I soon made some friends who appreciated me for who I was. I found that I was accepted in the Bible school and that each Bible student had his or her own individual reason for how he or she came to become a part of the Theology Institute.

I took my Bible training in theology seriously, and I found that I wanted to get good grades while in attendance at the school.

I found that the teaching was of excellent caliber, and I could sense the blessed Holy Spirit in the classrooms while I continued to learn about the great things of God. I especially appreciated Pastor Howard Paul Jennings, whom I came to appreciate as my favorite Bible instructor.

Not only was Pastor Jennings an excellent Bible professor with tremendous Bible knowledge, but he just exemplified being a man of God. I came to see that Pastor Jennings knew God in an amazing way.

This professor walked with God on a daily basis, and I was able to experience firsthand what it was like to learn the powerful teachings, doctrines, and revelations found in God's Word from a great man of God with authority. I recall that Pastor Jennings announced a three-day fast combined with prayer one day during our morning Bible chapel.

I decided to join in on the three-day fast, which I came to discover had good spiritual consequences for me. God was at work in my life as I attended the Bible school, and He had greater things for me to experience as I faithfully pursued the Lord in my life.

I remember a powerful revelation that came to me during one of my Gospel of John classes. Professor Ken Hendricks was sharing with the men and women present in the morning Bible school class that when the Holy Spirit came upon the virgin Mary, new life was conceived in her.

The spiritual truth ministered to me in a special way that day that my desire to have the life of God in my heart and life would come about by the power of the Holy Spirit. The blessed Holy Spirit working to bring about a quickening in my spiritual life had to be done through the wonderful works of the Spirit of God. I recall benefiting from going on a two-day fast before, and now while attending the Bible school, a three-day fast.

I decided to go on a five-day fast before the Lord, and I found that this helped me spiritually as well. I then began to read a book by Franklin Hall entitled *The Fasting Prayer,* which told about how God had worked in the lives of Christians embarking on protracted fasts, which included a fourteen-day fast, a twenty-one-day fast, and a forty-day fast.

I read about ordinary Christians seeing God performing miracles through their praying and fasting before the Lord. I made up my mind to go on a protracted fast to see God work mightily in my heart and life.

I continued to attend Union Theology Institute when I started on my lengthy fast. Everything was going fine on my fast, and then I remember standing up after I had bent down in the Institute's library to look for a book on the shelf. When I stood up, things went black momentarily in my mind; and from then on, I tried to be careful about getting up when I was on a protracted fast.

I wasn't inclined to end my fast over what I had experienced in the library. When I reached days sixteen to nineteen, I remember feeling a spiritual movement in my lower intestinal tract area that felt like something was spiritually moving inside of me. When I reached day twenty-two on the fast, I dropped off a completed assignment in the Theology Institute's library at night. A couple of my classmates saw me so skinny from fasting that they began to laugh at my thin appearance.

After the library incident, I became self-conscious about my physical condition. I decided to end my fast, but I knew from my reading in *The Fasting Prayer* that you need to be careful how you bring your fast to an end because you can injure yourself physically and cause yourself spiritual harm as well.

I decided to just have liquids like pink lemonade, hot chocolate, or a grapefruit drink from day twenty-three until day thirty. God was with me throughout the protracted fast, and I found that God was going to be with me in a greater way after completing my spiritual fast.

When I broke my protracted fast, I happened to be with a couple of friends who were interested in watching a football game together. Mark Fleming, Angie Caldwell, and I had agreed to get together to watch the game on television and have some snacks to go along with our viewing time.

I ended up throwing up from eating cookies and potato chips and drinking soda pop while watching the game. I discovered that the snacks and drink weren't the best things to be taking into my body purged from physical contaminants, chemicals, and poisons from food toxins that accumulate in our bodily systems, which need to be cleansed from impurities once in a while.

I discovered that the Holy Spirit had raised up in my life as a result of going on my protracted fast, causing me to experience a wonderful spiritual restoration in my heart and life like I had never experienced before. The living God of heaven and earth had quickened me spiritually, and I began to grow spiritually in my theological studies and in my relationship with God and man.

When I came back to my dorm room one day after the fast, I felt the Lord say, "Now, let's start marching as a soldier marching in the Lord's army." I had never sensed a revelation like that before, and I have come to recognize that it had to have come from the Lord Himself.

I was so encouraged by what God had done in my life as a result of my protracted fast that I decided to go on another one once the Bible school year was over.

The Ultimate Violation

That summer at the Scone's family home, I asked my mother, Jessica, if it was all right for me to borrow the tent and go up into the PumaPuma National Forest to camp out. Jessica responded in the affirmative, and I headed up to the mountains to have another visitation with God Himself through prayer and fasting. I found that I was only able to endure my spiritual camping trip for four days because of the cold days and nights that I was experiencing.

I found that the cold temperatures were becoming a distraction to me to spiritually concentrate on seeking God as I wanted and needed to do. I did find that out by the roadway, there was a hollow log that had wonderful-tasting springwater that I enjoyed.

I loaded up the car and headed back to Clover Valley to continue my fast at my parents' home. I had only water for the first four days of my fast, and then I drank different liquid drinks from day five to forty. When I reached day forty of my lengthy fast, I felt like I hadn't spiritually benefited from my fast because I was receiving nourishment from the various drinks I had during my fast. I decided to continue my fasting for the next seven days without any liquid drinks except for water.

For the next seven days, I persisted in wanting to experience the wonderful spiritual blessing of the Lord that comes from completing a fast. I was already a thin man, and now I was really skinny from the long fast that I had undertaken.

I remember the last night of my protracted fast and how I couldn't seem to get to sleep. When I heard a siren coming from a fire truck, I got up from my bed and walked over in the direction from which I had heard the siren. After returning to my bed to get some sleep, I found that my mind was active, which made me think of every restaurant that I had ever eaten at in Union before coming home for the summer break from the Theology Institute. I decided that I was going to break my protracted fast by having something to eat in the morning, especially since I had gone long enough without food.

I learned later that it was a good thing that I ended my fast when I did. My body was so thin as a result of my continuous fasting that it might have begun feeding on itself. I never consulted a physician before going on any one of my lengthy fasts.

I ended up having green grapes and cultured milk to help get my stomach acidic enzymes working again. I didn't have a powerful postfasting experience as I was hoping, but I believe the Lord wanted to reward me for my love for Him anyway.

I have come to the realization that He wants us to walk by faith as we seek His face, and not by sight nor feeling. The important thing for a Christian to do is to faithfully seek and serve the Lord and leave the spiritual rewards and results up to Him.

I returned to Union Theology Institute that fall to resume my great Bible training in theology. God would show Himself faithful to me throughout my Bible school days, and I found myself wanting to be used by the Lord as His servant in ministerial ways wherever I found open doors to minister for the Lord.

During my Theology Institute training, I was able to minister to souls during outside activities witnessing in the downtown area of Union, at the Banner Convalescent Center, on my personnel carrier routes whenever possible, and at the Golden Bells Chapel.

I was also able to do my own personal witnessing for the Lord wherever I was able to find someone interested in spiritual things in hopes of leading someone to Jesus Christ, the Savior of mankind. I found that I enjoyed attending Evangel Christian Fellowship Church, which had founded Union Theology Institute.

I had many good spiritual experiences while attending the church and being present in the Theology Institute classes, where I sensed the precious Holy Spirit's anointing presence. The anointing is the painting or coming upon of the Holy Spirit for the Lord's work as a chosen vessel. The anointing of the Holy Spirit enables a Christian believer to do things supernaturally for the Lord that he or she would not be able to do with their natural abilities.

The wonderful Holy Spirit's touch upon the pastors and Bible school instructors made the difference between receiving head knowledge in theological training, and experiential knowledge, which the Lord wants for all of His children to receive and experience daily.

I had fasted so long that I began to look like a person—sad to say—from a foreign country where there is a famine in the land. My mother, Jessica, wanted to take pictures of me in my super-thin physical condition. Jessica took a picture of me from a side position, and also one of my back to clearly show just how skinny I had become as a consequence of my protracted fast unto the Lord.

I believe that in a chosen fast, the Lord gives or calls a person for a specific reason and purpose. I also believe that if a Christian desires to seek after the Lord for some specific spiritual reason and purpose by giving himself or herself unto prayer and fasting, that the Lord will give that individual believer the desires of his or her heart.

I know that God is the giver of miracles and that He has great, good, and wonderful things in store for those who seek the Lord through prayer and fasting. I know that nothing is impossible for those Christians who dare to believe God for the miraculous in this day and hour. Many people do not believe in miracles today nor do they believe in a supreme deity; one day they will have to give an account of their lives to the supreme deity. "So then each of us shall give an account of himself to God" (Rom. 14:12 NKJV).

I know and believe that certain circumstances will not change on their own; they require Christians with pit-bull determination to see a miracle created and performed through their personal lives or in the lives of someone they know and love.

When I was attending Union Theology Institute, I learned about the Basic Youth Conflicts Seminar taught by instructor Bill Gothard, which was going to be in Seattle. My brother, Daniel, had told me about Bill's great Christian teachings, and so I decided that I would go and listen to this man of God teach on the principles of life for the Christian believer. I decided to make the trip to see Bill Gothard while he was in Seattle.

I was incredibly impressed with Bill's teachings and how life's principles were wonderfully explained, with illustrations to help and encourage those who desired to follow Christ's life principles to see God bring about the necessary positive changes in their lives.

I appreciated all of Bill's teachings, but I especially picked up on the subject matter where Bill mentioned that a change could be made to improve one's physical appearance if it were becoming a distraction to a Christian's focus on the Lord and the things of God.

Bill, at the time, was sharing about correcting a person's crooked teeth, which could be a distraction to his or her physical appearance, but I quickly applied the teaching to my nose, which led me to think that if something could be done to improve its appearance, I was willing to have it done.

I felt that my prominent nose was a distraction to my overall self-esteem, self-worth, and self-image as a Christian believer. I felt that my bulbous nose was holding me back from having a positive future in Christian ministry and marrying a wife who could join me in my Christian ministry.

I was experiencing some thoughts relative to being influenced by what I had seen glamorized on television. In the movies, it seemed to me glaringly obvious that Hollywood has chosen handsome men and beautiful women to act out their scripted roles in order to capture the viewing audiences. I have observed the emphasis on physical beauty that the entertainment industries select as America's beautiful people to lure the paying audience to the box office as well as purchase their movies on videocassettes and DVDs. I realize that I would have liked to be born with natural physical beauty admired by the people of the world, which in the order of things I wasn't blessed with the kiss or endowment of God by being physically attractive to beautiful women. I realize that physical beauty is really only skin deep, as many people have come to realize all over the world. I have come to recognize that God wanted me to accept my physical appearance just the way He created me to be.

On the other hand, I also thought God would think it was within reason and in good conscience to have corrective cosmetic surgeries that resulted in positive physical beauty enhancements if a person's physical unattractiveness became a detriment, distraction, or loss of God consciousness due to the person being obsessive over his or her physical appearance.

I recall going in to see the registrar at the Theology Institute one day to talk with him concerning how to determine what Christian woman to marry. Registrar Pastor Peter Sampson shared with me that he could have married five women and that each of them had their own unique special quality. He shared that when he met his wife, she had all the qualities of the other five women, and she had her own unique special quality as well. He let me know that I would have to decide for myself what qualities I was looking for.

I appreciated Dr. Sampson helping me with something to think about when it comes to finding the right woman to choose as my life's partner in marriage.

I remember a couple ladies at the Theology Institute that I had taken an interest in. One young, blond lady named Britney Langley caught my interest by the way she entered into worshiping the Lord during song and worship service. I thought she was a pretty lady who really loved the Lord,

THE ULTIMATE VIOLATION

but found that we had personality conflicts; I realized that I needed more maturity built into my character by the Lord.

I found that with the wonderful presence of the Holy Spirit working in my life, I was struggling with having a sensitive conscience regarding being honest about my reading assignments at the school and with feeling the importance of telling the truth in my personal relationships with men and women. I needed the Lord to strengthen me in the spirit of my character and break any bondages hindering the spirit of my mind.

I felt the need to tell the truth and to be honest before the Lord in my personal relationships. When I was given reading assignments by the different professors at the Bible school, knowing that honesty is the best policy, I wanted to honestly be able to say that I had completed my reading assignments. While in Bible school, I was experiencing an overactive conscience that was working overtime to keep me alert to my responsibilities before God and man. In my freshman year before going on my lengthy fast, I got hung up on reading the same word or phrases of words over and over to make certain I was reading my Bible assignments and the lessons that were given by my teachers in each class.

I was struggling with wanting to be an honest man and doing what my conscience was telling me to do. Britney was a gifted, straight-A student, and she found herself in a conflict with my personal struggles.

After having a good talk with Pastor Sampson regarding this problem, I felt free about moving on to reading groups of words in phrases instead of the individual words, which only hindered the spirit of my mind, making it feel like it had spiritual viruses, slowing my reading speed down to a snail's pace. God gave me the victory over this problem in my reading assignments with some good advice from Dr. Sampson.

I found myself telling Britney that I loved her by faith. Britney wasn't encouraged by my unusual way of telling her I loved her. I discovered that I wasn't positive I truly loved her as my future wife, and I found that the two of us had drifted apart during our tenure in the Theology Institute.

I took an interest in another young Christian lady who attended the Theology Institute, named Judy Clovis. I met Judy initially while the two of us were doing door-to-door witnessing as part of our outside activities that were required while attending Union Theology Institute.

At the time that we were witnessing together, I had taken an interest in Judy, who was a sophomore while I was a freshman, but I never asked her out until a number of months had passed by.

97

One day, I saw Judy in the Institute's library, and I found that I had taken a fancy to her with her attractive purple dress on that day. I happened to attend church with Judy one Sunday, and I was able to meet her parents later on. I had learned that it's good to see a potential wife in as many situations as possible before you ever take the plunge into a marriage relationship. I came to realize that it's a wise thing to not rush into getting married because many people who do, end up wishing they would have gotten to know their spouse a lot better before they said, "I do."

I discovered Judy's mother, Shirley Clovis, was overweight, and she had ongoing marital conflicts with her antagonistic husband. Nick Clovis was a nice man to me, but he was argumentative with his wife, Shirley. Nick seemed to always give his wife a hard time, and he proudly lacked any sensitivity and compassion toward Shirley.

I found that I liked Judy, who I could see was a rose between two thorns, but I decided not to marry her partly due to the discouraging marital tension and intense conflicts I witnessed in her home life.

I recall something that my sister Marlie had told me about a man trying to decide which one of two women he was seeing he should marry. The one woman was really homely, but she was talented and she could sing like a canary. The other woman was truly beautiful, but she couldn't sing. Finally, after some consideration, the man decided to marry the ugly woman who could really sing. Well, the two got married, and they ended up having their first night together on their honeymoon. In the morning, the husband looked over at his wife in bed, and seeing that his wife did not look any better to him after they tied the knot, he said, "Sing, baby, sing." I had gotten a kick out of hearing my sister's jest relative to one man's predicament in choosing the right wife as his life's soul mate.

I came to realize that I was influenced by the world's standards of beauty in wanting to change my physical appearance if I possibly was able to. I knew that I was self-conscious about my physical characteristics, but I wasn't always thinking about my looks, which was a good thing. The Lord was helping me with my physical appearance flaws, but I now realize that I had flaws in my thinking concerning my outward appearance that I should have continued to look to the Lord for help with.

I recognized that I had thought a lot about my physical looks, especially when I would become self-conscious whenever I looked at my Theology Institute album pictures. When I saw that they had included an embarrassing photo of myself during my freshman year, it really bothered me that they put in the worst of two pictures that the photographer had taken of myself. I found that my album picture was so awful to look at.

I found myself self-conscious throughout my remaining Theology Institute years. The negative picture experience of seeing myself in the freshman album made me that much more self-conscious and desirous to make a physical change if and whenever I was able to do so.

I graduated from the Union Theology Institute, and I continued to sense the presence of the Lord at work in my life postgraduation.

I discovered that I enjoyed traveling to see the Seattle Mariners baseball team, which is a major league professional team. The Seattle Mariners are the only professional major league baseball team in the Pacific Northwest.

Alex Tucker and I were friends and we were classmates in the Theology Institute; we liked traveling to the games whenever we could find time in hopes of seeing the professional team win the game. We found that the Mariners lost so many games that we had become discouraged with the team, and we would look forward to seeing the other team win. Alex and I got a kick out of telling others that we were going to watch the other team win the game.

We found that the ballgames were exciting to watch, especially when the New York Yankees, the Boston Red Sox, the Houston Astros with Nolan Ryan pitching, or the Oakland Athletics were in town.

I also liked to watch the University of Washington Huskies football team play on television. I came to enjoy going to see the semiprofessional Thunderbirds hockey team play a number of times whenever I could make the trip. To tell you the truth, I haven't gone to see the team play in years. although I discovered that the games could be really exciting.

I recall one Saturday afternoon when I had parked my William County personnel carrier shuttle some distance from the University of Washington Huskies football stadium while I was taking a break from driving. I had plans of walking over to the University of Washington's medical building during my break from driving when a nice couple on their way to the stadium inquired if I would like a free ticket to the Husky game.

Naturally I was truly receptive of the kind offer being made to me by the generous man, who went on to explain that their eleven-year-old son no longer liked to attend the games with his parents. I fully understood why I was being given a free gift of a lifetime, and I thoroughly enjoyed being a spectator at the great game on the gridiron with an upper-deck middle-of-the-field exceptionally fine viewing position. The Huskies won the game, and I was really grateful to such special people who had made it all possible for me to enjoy watching two top-caliber football teams battle it out on the playing field.

Although I enjoyed watching sports as a spectator, I recognized that being involved in the Lord's work was a greater calling than the pursuit of a sports dream while making big money from a lucrative contract.

I reminisced back to my teenage years, when I had read about Bob Feller, a tall, hard-throwing, fastball pitcher who played for the Yankees in 1939. I read how Bob would hold a shot put in his pitching hand for a period of time, and later when he held a baseball, it would feel as light as a feather in his hand. No wonder Bob was such an amazing fastball hurler during his prime years.

I also remember reading as an adult about Johnny Bench, who played for the Cincinnati Reds as an incredible catcher for years. I read that Johnny was able to throw a baseball from a squatting position up to 250 feet with pinpoint accuracy.

I also read that Johnny was able to hold seven baseballs in his large right hand. Unfortunately, I had inherited my mother's hands, and I was only able to hold four or five baseballs with all of my fingers on one hand hard at work to hold them all in place. I also learned about the sensational African American pitcher named Leroy Paige. Leroy had a nickname, "Satchel," that he liked to go by.

Satchel had amazing fastball speed, besides the other incredible pitches that he would use to surprise and catch the batters off guard who came up to face him at home plate. It was exciting to find out that the batters experienced real difficulties trying to hit his outstanding slew of pitches. I would have liked to see Satchel pitch as a spectator, especially during his prime years.

I would have enjoyed sitting next to my father watching Satchel Paige pitching against Bob Feller in that great game with Satchel at the helm at Sick's Stadium in Seattle. I discovered that Satchel had pitched in the major leagues when he was fifty-nine or sixty years old. I certainly was greatly impressed with all three of these incredible major league baseball players, who were inducted into baseball's famous hall of fame.

I also discovered that Satchel had pitched against Bob Feller in an exhibition charity game in Seattle, Washington, October 7, 1945. The pitching duel between the two sensational pitchers would have been a tremendous game to see along with my father, Benjamin, if only I had been born at an earlier time. I remember my father telling me about a game he had gone to where Satchel had been flown into a baseball stadium in a helicopter, and after he stepped out, he began warming up on the pitching mound. Now that would have been an exciting event to have seen sitting next to my dad in the stands.

I learned that Satchel had quite a variety of different names for his arsenal of incredible pitches, such as his own hesitation pitch and his sensational bee ball, which was his high-velocity fastball, to name just a couple of his amazing pitches. Satchel Paige's recipe for striking out opposing batters was laced with a mixture of the right ingredients to shut down even the best competitive baseball hitters. I would have liked to have watched and learned from Satchel, chief architect of such incredible and successful pitching talent as has ever put on a baseball uniform. Satchel was loved and admired by a great number of adoring fans for his pitching ability and delightful character. He truly enjoyed being a show-off, who he liked to portray in life. I realize that Satchel was a very interesting baseball player who had likable personality qualities, and he was highly honored by the fans who followed his baseball career. Satchel truly loved playing the great game of baseball, and he became a pitching legend.

Had I pitched professionally, I would have liked to have a 125-mile-an-hour fastball with a 109-mile-an-hour changeup. My pitching arsenal would have included names such as: hit this, the shocker, hot to trot, total surprise, lock bat, clean sweeper, don't even try, snail's pace, straight shooter, cry baby, talk to your bat, bat biter, brush-off pitch, I can't see you, reversible boomerang, thunderous momentum, no catch up, mouth stopper, maximum frustration, the tumbler, the drop-off, turn the key, acceleration pitch, guess who, I don't have all day, peekaboo, frost bat, chiller thriller, and don't even think about it.

I was able to acquire a brand-new intermediate Deering five-string banjo at a music store in Union. My Theology Institute classmate Judy Clovis was kind enough to purchase the banjo for me, and then I made payments to her until I had paid it off.

I wanted to learn to play the handsome, quality, intermediate banjo as soon as I could. I started out learning to play the banjo by playing chords with a plastic flat pick, and in time I was desirous to learn to play the bluegrass five-string picking style, with two metal picks and a plastic thumb pick. I have taken banjo lessons from a number of teachers through the years, and I have found that playing the banjo has helped me in so many ways. I had one banjo teacher, Matt Montegue, who had a six-thousand-dollar gold-plated Deering banjo, I have been able to sing and play my five-string banjo at Christian churches and at other Christian group gatherings for the Lord, as well as for personal entertainment for friends and family.

I have had the opportunity to hear some talented banjo pickers, including Butch Robbins, Earl Scruggs, Ralph Stanley, Bela Fleck, Sonny Osborne, and many other talented five-string banjo players at different times in the great state of Washington. I also was able to hear Bill Monroe at the Monroe Center in Seattle, playing his mandolin, and Mark O'Connor playing his amazing violin on a number of occasions at different times in Seattle.

My father, Benjamin, and I have enjoyed going to hear various bluegrass bands play some great-sounding music together over the years. I was especially impressed with Earl Scruggs playing his Gibson five-string banjo and his incredibly talented band that performed at the Bena Roya Hall in downtown Seattle.

I continued to attend the Evangel Christian Fellowship Church after I graduated from the Theology Institute, and I have continued working at William County Carrier.

I graduated with a degree in theology, and in time I began attending Sumpter Community College for some extra credits, which I needed to continue my college education. Sometime later, I also applied for the Pentecostal Bible Institute in Browerland, which was fully accredited, and found that I was accepted to attend the college in Browerland.

I discovered that the majority of the credits that I had earned at Union Theology Institute were accepted by the college I was interested in. My major was in Biblical literature, with a minor in counseling. God was continuing to bless me as I continued my college education and learned to play my five-string banjo.

I had moved from the dorm while attending Union Theology Institute and was able to find nice housing in the Banner District in Union. I paid rent for housing while attending the Theology Institute and later when I attended different classes at the Pentecostal Bible Institute in Browerland.

I remember one summer when I had gone home to the Scone family home in Clover Valley. Randell Wikum had come down for a visit, and he needed a place to stay since he and Carol weren't doing very well in their marriage relationship.

One day I, Benjamin, and Randell decided to go up Feather Creek to do some fishing. I recall how Randell was engrossed in his fishing when I proceeded to sneak up behind his location across an open, dry-weed field. Randell was just below the open field's bank, situated on the north side of Feather Creek, which was flowing eastward.

As I was creeping across the field, I was doing my best to stay low so that Randell couldn't catch a glimpse of me coming from behind. When I felt that I was in the right proximity to Randell's fishing position, I lit a black-cat firecracker and flicked it in his direction with a perfect finger toss. It lit right behind Randell, and it exploded with a loud cracking pop.

Randell was caught completely off guard, and being startled, he said, "Kurtess, would you grow up?"

I was pretty pleased with myself that I had surprised Randell with a firecracker in good sport.

Later, when we were back at the Scone family residence, Randell snuck a baby-finger firecracker of his own through the bathroom window where I was drying off from taking a bath. The baby-finger firecracker fizzled, and it didn't explode with a payback explosion as Randell was hoping for. Later, when Randell was out, I short-sheeted his bed and put cornflakes in his sheets.

Unfortunately, Randell detected something peculiar about the bed he was going to sleep in and was able to thwart my mischievous plans of giving him a hard time out of good fun.

I recognize that Randell was a good sport at times throughout his marriage to my sister Carol.

When I went back to Union, I found that I liked to counsel people one-on-one in my personal relationships. I enjoyed sharing with my friends Christian doctrines, words of wisdom, and knowledge through counseling insights, and counseling with words of encouragement to friends and acquaintances that I knew.

I recall witnessing in downtown Union. I saw an African American man on the sidewalk who came up to me and my witnessing partner, Chris, saying, "I know what you're down here for." He went on to tell us that on the dollar bill, it says, "In God we trust, and as long as I have that dollar bill, I trust in God."

I have come to realize that there are a lot of characters in this world who need evangelizing for Christ Jesus, but they are too egotistically proud and wrapped up in their own philosophical head games, having preconceived notions and ideas about trusting in God, knowing God, and how to rightly live for God. The Lord expects us to walk humbly before Him with humility of heart and mind.

God says, "He has shown you, O man, what is good; And what does the Lord require of you But to do justly, To love mercy, And to walk humbly with your God?" (Mic. 6:8 NKJV).

I met my friend Greg Danielson while working at William County as a personnel carrier driver. When I was attending Union Theology Institute, I applied for a job with William County Carrier as a personnel carrier operator, and I was hired by the company in the eighties to drive a carrier for them. Greg had approached me out in the carrier site one day and inquired if we could get together sometime for lunch to talk. I had taken a course on pastoral care and counseling while attending the Pentecostal Bible Institute and a counseling course at Union Theology Institute.

I tried to be a personal friend and a positive source of encouragement to Greg, who seemed to have some legitimate problems in his personal life. The things that bothered him had caused a great deal of emotional suffering for Greg.

I would look for ways to offer my friend good advice and wisdom that he might be able to apply to his personal life and in his relationships with women.

I came to see Greg as an immature Christian, who had a lot of questions without solid answers that would bring him legitimate relief, actual help, and genuine satisfaction that God could fulfill his needs. Greg had plenty of questions that he liked to ask me or a friend who would come along for a lunch or for a dinner get-together. Greg didn't always seem to have answers to his own questions, and he enjoyed playing the devil's advocate with me and others. Greg communicated to me that God had passed him over when it came to having brains and good looks.

One day he admitted to me that he felt like he was a seven on the looks category and he wasn't a good communicator with the ladies. I tried to encourage Greg by providing some good advice on what he could talk about with any potential date he might encounter. Greg felt like the women weren't giving him enough time to get to know him. Once they found out Greg was a part-time carrier driver, he wasn't successful at securing a date with any women.

I continued to be a positive source of encouragement to Greg throughout the many years of our friendship. I had learned that Greg was able to have a friendship with two women who found that they appreciated his friendship with them. One he played tennis with, and the other he would get together with to talk to as a friend. Greg and I experienced the following together: having lunches and dinners together, playing tennis, going bowling, playing chess, competing in running against each other, golfing, arm wrestling, attending sports events, attending a church service or Christian concert, and being on a double date.

Greg communicated to me that he had a thousand questions for God when he would get to heaven. Greg found that he liked to ask me for the answers to questions that he felt there are no answers to.

I believed that God already provided the answers for us as recorded in the Bible, and the Holy Spirit can give us answers that we may be struggling with intellectually and emotionally.

Greg found himself in competition with me in key areas of his personal life relative to sports, spirituality, and relationships with women. He told me that he believed he was a better tennis player than I was, and I related to Greg that we should let the outcome of the games prove who was the better player. Throughout the years, Greg worked hard to defeat me in tennis and in other games of competition where we competitively participated against one another, but in the final analysis, I defeated my friend Greg in more sporting events than he won. When it came to spiritual matters, I could see that Greg felt that God should be making provisions for him as a father would provide for his son. Greg shared with me that he had been a Christian for thirty-five years. I could also see that Greg had areas in his life that he needed to work on first in order for him to find the right woman of his dreams. Greg felt that he was missing out on a lot of things that God had promised in His Word, that He hadn't provided the fulfillment of His promise for him. Greg didn't appreciate waiting for God to answer his prayers, especially when it came to finding a good woman to marry.

I recall one Sunday night on which Greg and I attended Westgate Chapel, a good Christian church in Edmonds. Following the church service, Greg and I decided to go to Denny's twenty-four-hour restaurant before traveling to our respective homes.

Greg and I pulled out separately from the church parking lot, and each of us was determined to beat the other at arriving first at Denny's. Greg had gotten an early lead in his '77 Chevy Vega. I was surprised to see Greg sitting at a stop sign waiting for the southbound traffic to clear when I pulled up in my '75 Chevy Vega on the right shoulder next to the concrete bulkhead. I could see that Greg did not look in my direction when he started to make a right turn directly into my bronze metallic Vega.

I had assumed that before Greg ever began to make his right turn, he would look over to his right and clearly see that I was sitting there ready to make my right-hand turn also. I discovered that Greg never knew I had snuck in on his right side before he ran into my car's left front bumper. Discovering that he had run into my Chevy Vega, Greg backed up to allow me to pull out first in our race to Denny's.

When we went inside of Denny's restaurant, we both had ourselves a long hearty laugh together over our amusing accident. I apologized to Greg for what I had done to cause the accident in the first place, and Greg was forgiving of his friend for pulling up and moving out of the clearly marked white boundary lines where a single car is permitted to drive. I was considered outside of the boundary as far as the law is concerned, and I thank the good Lord that Greg didn't hold it against me for the crinkled wheel well of his '77 Chevy Vega. My '75 Chevy Vega had the black rubber stripe pulled loose on my left front bumper; I was able to glue it back flush onto my silver bumper, which caused it to match the car body.

One day a passenger wanted to know if I could lead him in a prayer after I had shared the love of God with him on my personnel carrier. The man's name was James Salvador, and he gave his life to the Lord as I led him in a sinner's prayer right on the carrier coach.

James and I were alone on the personnel carrier after I made a stop with my carrier coach on Island Summit Way on Kismet Island during a winter snowstorm in 1986. I didn't have chains on my carrier, and when

I tried to continue to drive my carrier route, I found that I wasn't able to get my carrier vehicle to move.

Without chains on the tires, I didn't have any traction to move the heavy carrier in the snow. After I had placed some ground black coal from a plastic container on the carrier under my tires, I still wasn't able to continue driving my carrier route. I had made a crucial mistake in stopping my carrier coach on the hill after someone had rung the chime chord. I realized I should have made it to the top of the hill before stopping.

On a separate occasion, I invited an African American passenger, Bill Henderson, to come with me to a Westgate Chapel Church service to hear the evangelist James Robinson preach. Bill came with me to the evangelistic Christian service, and he gave his life to the Lord Jesus. Bill was new in town, and he had to wait for his baggage to arrive the next day at the Greyhound Bus station.

I took the now-Christian man home with me, and Bill was so appreciative to me for my Christian kindness to take in a complete stranger for food and shelter. The next day, I was able to provide a ride for Bill to the bus station so that he could get his baggage.

God was using me for his Christian service and ministry, and I looked for ways that I might be able to serve the Lord by bringing people to Christ Jesus who were interested and open to receiving Him as Lord and Savior.

I recall going to a tae kwon do martial arts center in the Brocket District with my carrier driver friend Lynn McConnel in hopes of being able to see a martial arts demonstration.

I had been able to watch a martial arts demonstration at the center before alone. We already had lunch at the Kings Table Buffet, and now we wanted to see a good demonstration of martial arts between a couple of well-trained individuals or by someone working out by himself to improve his martial arts with precision body skills, finesse, and power.

Lynn had told me that he had a black belt in karate, but he didn't want to tell the martial arts instructor at the training center about his black belt status. The instructor turned out to be a nine grandmaster in tae kwon do, and instead of letting Lynn and I see a martial arts demonstration, he began demonstrating on us some of his simple moves that would stop an opponent in a hurry. The demonstration being performed on the two carrier operators was felt with unpleasant pain.

Lynn and I walked away from the martial arts center unhappy with the demonstration being applied directly to our unsuspecting physical bodies. I was able to attend an actual martial arts demonstration after that day at the tae kwon do martial arts center, although the two carrier drivers were disappointed with what we had personally experienced at the hands of the nine grandmaster.

One day, Lynn and I drove from the Rolland carrier site, the only personnel carrier site of the William County Carrier Company, to the Brocket District for lunch. We decided to go to a pizza parlor for their all-you-can-eat pizza during the lunch hour. Lynn and I were enjoying eating the toppings off each of our slices of pizza and placing the crust made of dough onto a brown plastic tray.

After consuming a lot of good-tasting pizza toppings between the two of us, the stack of pizza dough was growing higher with each topping slice devoured. After a good deal of toppings had disappeared at Lynn's and my table, the manager came over to have a talk with Lynn. He told him that he was going to have to stop eating the pizza the way he was doing, or the manager was going to call the police. Lynn told the manager that he was going to have to do what he had to because we weren't going to stop eating the way we were.

The manager gave Lynn the money back for his order, and he never said a thing to me, who had been eating my pizza the same way as Lynn. I had learned how to eat the toppings off of the pizza from watching my landlord, Charlene Spencer, a senior citizen Christian, eat her pizza one day.

Lynn was unhappy with me for not speaking up to the manager as he had done. When the manager was confronting Lynn regarding the way he was eating his pizza, I remained as quiet as a church mouse sitting at the table. I was stopped in my tracks from eating any more pizza slices when I heard the manager confronting Lynn about the way he was eating his pizza.

We found our enjoyable lunch experience brought to a halt by the manager. It was a total surprise and seemed like overkill of our choice of how we wanted to eat our pizza. The two friends left Godfather's Pizza before the police were ever called—or at least before they ever arrived.

I had met my friend Greg before I had come to know Lynn through our carrier association. I came to see Lynn as an intellectual sort and a reasoning type of a person, who appreciated having a dialogue with me by intellectualizing and reasoning his way to understanding God and the ways of God. Lynn told me that he saw Greg as a baby Christian with a big diaper, who was beating up on God by complaining all the time about why He wasn't meeting his individual needs.

Lynn had grown disgusted with Greg's negative thinking and continuous complaining about his unsuccessful life. Lynn got to the place that he didn't want to be around Greg because of his negative perspective of not seeing positive results in his life. When Greg, Lynn, and I were having lunch one day at the King's Table Buffet, Lynn told Greg, "You're going to hell."

Naturally Greg thought Lynn had misjudged him regarding his relationship with God and his eternal destiny in the future.

At the Rolland carrier site, Lynn had some more words for Greg. He said, "If I wasn't a Christian, I'd beat the crap out of you."

Greg didn't have words to say to Lynn at this point, but he did want to talk to me. I understood that Greg and Lynn only wanted to have an ongoing friendship with me and definitely not with each other.

I found that I had appreciated my relationship with Greg over the years, but I recognized that Greg did have some erroneous thinking about his relationship with God and with women.

I continued to try to encourage my friend, even when my words of wisdom and positive advice didn't seem to make any difference.

Greg liked to inquire of me what I would do if I got married and my wife packed on three hundred pounds and didn't want to exercise to shed those unwanted pounds. *What if she was in a car accident, and you couldn't have sexual relations anymore?*

Greg liked to think of the worst scenarios concerning the marriage relationship with the opposite sex that he could think of to get my perspective. I would provide Greg with what I considered words of wisdom from God's perspective and what would be a good answer that Greg might think was the right way to view a committed marriage relationship.

I would remind Greg that a man should honor his marriage vows for better or for worse, in sickness and in health; he should remain committed to his wife.

Greg would say, "But what if you're not happy in the relationship? Would God expect you to stay in an unhappy relationship?"

I could see the importance of remaining faithful before God to your loving spouse regardless of whether she was in perfect physical health and wasn't as physically attractive as she was on the day you married her.

Greg had experienced so many negative circumstances and rejections from women throughout the years that he had developed a defeatist attitude in his relationship with them.

I picked up on the fact that Greg had experienced so many rejections from his dating proposals with the opposite sex that his words came across as fatalistic, defeatist, and critically negative.

I had been dealing with Greg for years regarding his reoccurring and seemingly endless negative thinking about the insincere things that even Christian women are guilty of committing. Greg had been at Christian churches and dances where he would ask a nice Christian lady to go out for coffee, to lunch, to a concert, or to play tennis.

Greg had so many women who had given their phone numbers to him only to say when he called later that they were busy or that they had a boyfriend. Greg couldn't understand why Christian women wouldn't merely tell him up front when he initially asked them out that they weren't interested or that they had a boyfriend. He had grown distasteful with Christian women who he felt should be honest in their relationships with men, and yet they had shown him that they didn't have good character qualities to be honest with men up front.

I tried sincerely to inform Greg that many women, because of their emotional nature, can't seem to tell the would-be suitor who may not be the man of their dreams that they have other plans, commitments, or a boyfriend. If they have a boyfriend, what are they doing in a Christian singles' group?

Greg questioned the Christian women's motives as well when it came to the art of honest communication with men. I found that Greg had negatively questioned me about women for so long that I thought I would provide Greg an interesting situation concerning the opposite sex for him to answer. I thought that I would give Greg a good taste of his own medicine for a switch.

It had become apparent to me that Greg had more than enough negative relationship situations to question me about, which always had a fatalistic spin or twist that could lead to a negative conclusion. No matter what positive answer I would provide for Greg, it seemed he had another negative question to ask me about after I answered that one.

So after years of continuous negative questions, I inquired of Greg what he would do in this situation. My own worst scenario went like this: "What if you had met the woman of your dreams, who had a beautiful figure, measured up in every way that you would want in a woman, was interested in sports, and could play tennis?" This was pretty important for him.

I let Greg think that the woman I had described would make him happy as his wife, but she had one problem. I had brought Greg to the pinnacle of thinking his potential wife only had one flaw, and now he was ready with a twist of his own, directed at Greg to answer for a change.

I was now ready to share with Greg the big punch line to see if he would marry this wonderful woman who only had one difficult condition to overcome. I said to Greg, "She doesn't have a vagina. Would you marry her?" Greg answered me in the negative. Greg felt that the woman he would marry needed to have the standard pieces of equipment that had made her a person of interest to him.

One day, Greg and I debated an important issue between ourselves, and I decided to let Greg read what the Bible had to say about the matter. Greg liked to play the devil's advocate when he debated or argued with me concerning spiritual subjects, social issues, relationship matters, political parties, and sports. Greg liked to feel that he could debate me with confidence regarding whatever the subject happened to be.

When I showed Greg the Bible passage that I believed would settle the matter, thinking that Greg would concede that my points were in line with God's thoughts on the matter, Greg boldly said to me, "I don't care what you say. I don't care what the Bible says. I've got to live in this world."

I was surprised to hear Greg utter those words to me, and I told Greg that he wasn't a Christian. Greg was hurt to hear my quick evaluation of his relationship to Jesus Christ, but I felt that Greg was definitely in the wrong to ever make a declaration of total disregard for what God had stated as eternal truth in the Holy Bible; His Word will never be revoked by the one true God, who can never lie.

I have come to realize that there may be other professing Christians who feel the same as Greg does, but have never voiced their convictions that they need to conform to the world in order to survive in this cold, cruel world. Jesus told his believers that He has overcome the world by His faith, and every Christian can absolutely with God's help overcome this world by using his or her faith.

I recall a time when I had a sleeper on my personnel carrier shuttle out at Coffer Community College south of Union. I was driving my carrier route when I reached my destination at the Coffer Community College parking lot designated carrier terminal. I observed the sleeping customer lying down on the seats in the back carrier section. He wasn't getting up as expected, and so I thought that I would help him to wake up in order to leave my carrier coach. I suspected the sleeper was intoxicated and that he wouldn't be fazed by what I had to say over the intercom system. I took hold of the microphone and said, "If anyone is caught sleeping on this carrier, they will be shot on sight."

To my surprise, the man quickly got up and wanted out the door of the carrier. I obliged the man's sudden interest in getting off of my personnel carrier, and I opened the door to let the client step off of my large motor personnel carrier. I found that the sleeper was no longer a sleepy passenger, and he eagerly left my carrier coach with haste.

I discovered that I could play the lip trumpet over my intercom system on my carrier shuttles. One early morning I was driving a William County Carrier Express shuttle route from Hoover Beach to downtown Union. As I was driving my carrier route, I discovered that one of the elderly passengers on my carrier was going to retire soon. I made an announcement over the intercom system requesting that the customers join me in singing, "We Wish You a Happy Good Year" along the melody of "We Wish You a Merry Christmas."

After the passengers and I sang the song for the retiring senior citizen, I played the Merry Christmas melody with my lip trumpet. When I had finished blowing into the microphone with the use of my lips playing the melody, the passengers on my carrier shuttle began to applaud. I continued to safely drive my personnel carrier, stopping at each appropriate stop along the route.

When I eventually stopped at Eighth and Executive in downtown Union, a tall African American man came walking up front and said to me, "I've been playing the trumpet for sixteen years. You sounded like you were playing the horn."

I accepted the compliment from the considerate passenger as an acknowledgement of my lip-trumpet playing talents. I have enjoyed playing the lip trumpet for my clients during the Christmas season with a variety of Christmas songs that are the customers' favorites.

I also transported schoolkids to their respective schools while driving for William County Carrier. One hot summer day in June, I had an African American boy who was about to get off of the personnel carrier shuttle. I recall saying to the cute little elementary child, "Now, don't you catch cold out there."

The small boy looked directly at me and said, "Yeah, right." He then proceeded to step off the carrier.

I liked to communicate with my passengers by saying, "Have a good day!" or "Have a good night." I frequently shared a friendly smile with my passengers to try to make them feel welcome on my carrier shuttles.

One day I communicated to a senior citizen woman passenger who happened to carry a cane, "I see you're raising cane." I followed my comment with, "One good thing about cane—it makes you able."

The female customer let me know that she liked that. I liked to tell passengers and other carrier drivers the Willy Nelson joke. I'd say, "Have you heard the sad news about Willy Nelson? I was listening to the news today, and they said that he got run over."

The passengers would say something like, "Oh no, really? Was he killed?" I liked to play along with the person as long as I could. I would then give them the punch line that Willie was playing on the road again.

Some of the people when I provided the punch line would catch on to the fact that it was just a joke. One senior carrier driver had been leaning out into the aisle to hear what I had to say about Willy Nelson's death. When I told Jason the punch line, he sat back in his front passenger seat and acted like he didn't care to hear anything more that I had to say. The Willy Nelson joke was a good attention-getter. I found that having something humorous, kind, and considerate to say can go a long way to brighten a passenger's day.

I inquired of my customer friend Larry, who worked for the Morris Parking Company with Avista Transportation, if he had caught the fight at the candy store. I told Larry up front that the sucker got licked. Larry acted all interested in hearing the gory details of the big fight that I was telling him about, and by the way I described the fight, it must have sounded to Larry like the person getting licked had experienced a through thrashing. Larry kept pressing me for more details of the contest between the two opponents, and I kept repeating that the sucker got licked at the candy store. Larry wanted to know what candy store, and so I provided the name of a store that Larry was familiar with in Union—Bristol's, a pharmacy drugstore.

Time and time again, I would repeat the same line about the sucker getting licked at the candy store. Larry kept insisting on hearing the bloody description of the struggle, and I repeated over again the same line of the sucker getting licked. I let Larry know that that was the fight. The sucker got licked. When it was obvious that Larry wasn't catching onto the fact that it was a corny joke that I had told different passengers over the years, I finally let Larry know that it was just a joke. The sucker had been licked at the candy store. What a fight it was.

Having to repeat myself to my customer friend Larry reminds me of when I told a friend about two parrots named Pete and Repeat sitting on a fence together. I told my friend, "Pete flew away, so who was left?" He answered, "Repeat." So I repeated the same scenario over again exactly the way I described it the first time. Once again he said, "Repeat." I have found that not everybody catches on to the funny scenario the first time you tell it to them; it is only meant for a joke.

One day a talented young lady named Jackie McPhearson, who was on her way home to Kismet Island, rode my carrier coach. Jackie informed me that she attended Cornish Art Institute, which I discovered was Cornish College of the Arts on Capitol Hill in Seattle, Washington.

She graciously gave me an invitation to come to see her perform in a play in which she sang and acted like Julie Andrews had in the movies. I was truly impressed with Judy's singing and acting abilities as revealed during the evening performance.

Jackie had some fun with me by telling me some corny jokes while I drove my carrier route. Jackie said, "Let me hear you spell silk."

I responded, "S-I-L-K" one letter at a time.

"What do cows drink?"

I responded, "Milk."

Jackie said, "Wrong. Cows drink water. Calves drink milk."

I thought that was a pretty good joke.

Jackie said, "Let me hear you say *roast*."

I responded, "Roast."

Jackie said, "Let me hear you say *boast*."

I said, "Boast."

Jackie said, "Let me hear you say *almost*."

I responded, "Almost."

Then Jackie said, "What do you put in a toaster?"

I responded, "Toast."

Jackie said, "No, you put bread in, and you get toast back."

I was impressed with Jackie's jokes. She had caught me during her carrier ride, and I found that I was able to catch other people on the same humorous jokes over the years.

I recall getting together with a nice couple of carrier operators who worked at William County Carrier. The couple were married, and they wanted to share a business plan with me; they thought I might be interested in joining to make some extra money outside of the carrier company. Rex and Cathy Bernard were kind enough to take time out of their day to share with me what they hoped would be a win-win proposition that could turn out to be a successful business opportunity.

I arrived late at the Denny's restaurant, and I informed them that I didn't have long to spend with Rex and Cathy because I had another meeting to go to. Later in their workweek, Rex told me that he had shared the business opportunity with the waiter after I had left. The waiter told Rex that he had a daughter and that he had come into some money.

Rex assumed that he had come into thirty-five thousand dollars which was a figure that came to his mind as a waiter working at the restaurant, and he kept trying to sell the waiter on the business plan. After sharing with the waiter, Rex could tell he wasn't catching fire on the business. He then inquired how much money the waiter had come into. The waiter told him forty-two million dollars. The waiter had waited on this man for nine years, and he never knew that he had that kind of money.

Rex told me the same man who gave the waiter forty-two million had done the same for four other people. When I was driving home after hearing Rex's story about the good fortune of the waiter, I thought to myself, *Can you believe that? That is truly a human-interest story.*

I found myself thinking that here I was working to make a living and this man has all this money just given to him. When I inquired of the manager at Denny's restaurant regarding the story of the waiter coming into a financial bonanza of forty-two million, I found out the story was true.

I asked if the waiter was going to continue to work at Denny's, and the manager told me yes. The last time I followed up to see if the waiter was still working at Denny's, I found that the restaurant had closed down its business.

I made my usual client pickup at Seventh Avenue and Royal Diamond Street in Union in order to drive my 777 carrier shuttle route out to Polo and Collard one Saturday evening. I drove my southbound trip all the way out to the city of Collard, and when it came time to pull into the Collard Carrier Center, I observed a vehicle in front with its left turn signal on. I assumed the driver would continue turning into the parking lot of the east side of the carrier center without stopping, but instead I was caught off guard when the vehicle held up for an oncoming car some distance ahead.

I had to make a sudden stop to avoid hitting the vehicle in front of my carrier; and when I braked, an elderly woman, anticipating my stop at the Collard Carrier Center, fell backward onto the hard floor of the carrier. The woman hit her head in the aisle of the coach, and a couple of men helped her up, where she sat down in the first seat across from me.

After the passengers had gotten off the coach at the carrier center, I was able to talk with the lady to inquire how she was. At the time, she thought she was all right, but as she felt the back of her head, she wasn't quite so sure. I inquired if she was willing to remain on the carrier so I could continue to make certain she was going to be perfectly fine.

The woman agreed to remain on the carrier shuttle, and I was able to monitor my passenger by listening to the things she was saying. During the course of the carrier route, I heard the woman say that she didn't know how she was going to be and she was going to have her son take her to the hospital to be checked out. When I heard my female passenger saying these words of uncertainty concerning her well-being, I knew I was going to need to fill out an accident report when I returned back to the Rolland Carrier site.

At the end of the carrier line, I had a male passenger with a brown trench coat come walking up to the front of the carrier and ask me if I saw who had taken his bag. I could tell the man was upset about his missing bag, however large, and I told the man that I never saw anyone take his bag.

The man continued to search around his seating area until he came up another time to inquire of me what my ID number was that was issued to me by the carrier company. I told the man, "W-I-L-L-I-A-M."

The Ultimate Violation

I could tell the angry man was not amused by my answer. The man had gotten off the carrier only to return a short time later for another vigorous search of the carrier coach for his bag, followed by one occasion when he slammed his fist into the passenger window, whereby he broke it with a fierce blow.

Finally, I had the presence of mind to inquire of the frustrated and fuming man where he had gotten on the personnel carrier. The steaming passenger responded to me that he had gotten on at Fifth and Cellar, which I knew was in downtown Union.

I informed the man that I took over the carrier route at Seventh and Royal Diamond, which is south of downtown Union. I knew the angry passenger was doing his level best to hold me responsible for his missing bag, and I was not going to accept responsibility for the man's missing possession. The male passenger admitted to me that he had fallen asleep on my carrier coach, and I knew the passenger was responsible for his own missing bag.

I was able to continue my concerned conversation with the woman who had fallen on my personnel carrier each time the angry man got off my carrier after making repeated searches for his lost bag.

The final time the irate passenger exited my carrier coach, the injured woman said, "Man, he is scary."

I heard the female passenger say that she was concerned that he might have a gun. I made the important phone call to report the accident of the woman falling on my carrier and also the man breaking the window while on my coach.

Once the angry man had finally left from searching the coach for his missing bag, I took the opportunity to feel the back of the woman's head where she had made contact with the carrier floor. I was surprised to feel a good-sized bump on her head, and I realized it was probably best that she have it checked out by a doctor, especially at her age. The woman said she knew of a woman who had gotten a bump on her head and ended up dying. This was not something I wanted to hear, but she had related to me that she was going to have her son take her to the hospital. I drove my remaining passenger back to the Collard Carrier Center, where she stepped off my carrier shuttle.

As I drove my 777 carrier shuttle route back to downtown Union, and subsequently Route 999 to the Mandalay District, thought about the angry man who had gotten upset regarding his missing bag. He was insistent on holding me responsible for his missing possession. As I contemplated the possibility of the angry passenger waiting for me at the end of the line, which is the terminal for the last stop on my 777 carrier shuttle route, I became concerned the man could be hiding behind a tree with a gun.

These concerned thoughts were going through my mind as I sat on my personal carrier by Dickens Park in the dark of night. Later, when I came slowly driving up to the carrier terminal at the end of my 777 carrier shuttle route in Collard, I was peering at the trees to see if the man could be lurking behind one of them with a loaded gun, armed and dangerous. When the man was nowhere in sight, I turned off my carrier shuttle to rest my head on my crossed arms resting on the steering wheel.

A couple of minutes before I was to begin my next trip into downtown Union on the 777 carrier shuttle route, I heard three loud pounding sounds on the driver's side window.

I immediately looked out the window, and when I didn't see anyone, I quickly looked into my driver side mirror only to see the same angry man walking back down Twenty-Seventh Avenue NE away from my carrier coach. I was startled by what had just transpired with the still-fuming passenger pounding with his fist on the side window. When I made the loop back over to 273rd and Twenty-Ninth Avenue NE and came to a stop at the red stop sign, I witnessed the man with the brown trench coat walking away from my carrier location with his back turned toward me.

As I reflected on the three hard poundings on my side window, I came to interpret the man's pounding message as "Bang, Bang, Bang, I could have shot you while you slept."

I never saw the man ever again on one of my carrier routes. It certainly was an unusual experience during my personnel carrier-driving career that had given me a good scare.

One night I was able to get the night off from driving three trips on my regular route 456 shuttle from downtown Union to Hoover Beach, and on the return, two trips from Hoover Beach to downtown Union. Later on, I would drive two round-trips on two separate late-night service carrier routes leaving from Sixth Avenue and Frontier Street in downtown Union. Route 876 left downtown at 1:45 a.m., and Route 879 left from Sixth and Frontier at 3:45 a.m.

When I returned to work on my regular carrier route, I discovered that a homeless African American man had waited for my carrier shuttle to show up at Twelfth Avenue and Capella Street. When my carrier shuttle

456 happened to show up at the carrier stop, the homeless man remained standing outside at the carrier stop. The substitute driver opened the door to inquire if the passenger was going to get on the coach. The man said he was waiting for me to show up. The carrier driver responded, "Hotel Kurtess. I know him." The patient homeless man was disappointed to learn that I had taken the night off from work and that he would have to wait for another night to catch up with the caring carrier driver.

I had attracted quite a number of homeless individuals who looked forward to riding with me on my late-night carrier service. Unfortunately for me, not all of my fellow carrier drivers appreciated my kindness and hospitality toward the homeless—and for good reason. A number of drivers felt like I was setting a bad example that they, too, would have to follow. From my perspective, I was showing acts of caring compassion toward people who didn't have a home of their own. My late-night carrier service became known as a moving motel on wheels, and unfortunately my carrier coach had unpleasant odors that other, respectable night riders didn't appreciate.

My carrier was well-known for its hospitality motel service to the homeless. I discovered that the carrier supervisor who oversaw the late-night service from downtown Union was fully aware of my viewpoint regarding providing a helpful, comfortable seat to people less fortunate than others.

Melody Paradise had taken a special interest in me as her personnel carrier driver in Collard. Melody, a kindhearted senior citizen, had a couple of hobbies: writing poetry, and taking pictures of carrier drivers and other things that she found especially of interest to her.

One Saturday, I showed Melody a childhood picture of myself and my good friend Treat Munson sitting together on the couch inside of the Scone family house in Clover Valley, before we went out trick-or-treating on Halloween night.

I inquired if Melody could have my picture enlarged inside Bristol's Drugstore nearby the Collard Carrier Center. I jokingly informed Melody that I was the one dressed as a clown with my girlfriend as the two sat right close to one another holding hands.

Melody let me know that she was willing to have my picture developed, and she also had a copy made for herself because she liked the cute picture. Later, when Melody was coming up onto the personnel carrier on the lift operation for people with walkers such as herself, she said to me, "Why didn't you hang onto her? She is so beautiful." I responded to Melody's surprising question that I had held onto my girlfriend all of these years. Melody didn't understand exactly what I meant by my answer, since she knew that I now had my lovely wife, Lorena Scone.

I eventually was able to provide Melody the hidden secret of what I meant by telling her that I had held onto my childhood girlfriend all of these years because I was not the boy dressed up as the clown in the picture, but instead I was the boy dressed up as Treat Munson's girlfriend. Melody finally understood the mystery of the cute couple sitting on the sofa in the Scone's family dwelling. As Melody reflected on my explanation of the couple in the picture, she thought it was such a good story to hear.

I recall a couple women I had taken an interest in after graduating from Union Theology Institute. One blond named Jennifer Berg was an attractive woman who I thought had a nice-looking nose. Jennifer was a good Christian lady who was interested in serving the Lord in the ministry along with her future husband. Jennifer was good at working with small children in day care, and I found that she was caring and sensitive concerning the things of the Lord.

Jennifer found herself comparing herself with her sister, who was already married and had children. Jennifer thought that I would make a good addition to the Berg family by marrying her. Jennifer and I liked to talk about the Lord and Christian counseling, listen to music, attend church together, and get together for lunch or dinner engagements. It was sometime later that I got to meet Jennifer's parents, who had come out to visit their daughters in Union.

I discovered that Mr. Berry Berg had an ugly, large nose that gave me major concerns regarding marrying Jennifer. I balked at the prospects of marrying Jennifer because I thought if we had children, there was a good possibility that the child would end up with a prominent nose too.

I also took an interest in an attractive woman from the Philippines named Phoebe Philomena, who was a passenger on one of my personnel carrier routes. One day I invited Phoebe to go with me to the Evangel Christian Fellowship Church in Union. I found out that Phoebe had grown up in a very conservative, traditional, religious home with her parents in the Philippines. She was living with her father at the time in south Union. Her mother had remained in the Philippines, where she was able to take care of their crops with the hired servants. I shared with Phoebe where I could see that the religious church she was attending was not in agreement with the Bible, and Phoebe found herself listening to what I had to share with her concerning her traditional religious church.

She wasn't accustomed to hearing the Biblical teachings I was telling her about in her church. Phoebe told me at a later time that what I had shared with her concerning the ritualistic traditional church she had attended for most of her life had hurt her when I told her the different ways their teachings were in contradiction with the Bible.

After I picked her up for church in my car, we drove out together to the Evangel Christian Fellowship Church service. I had heard that evangelist Peter Youngren was going to be at the church that night, and I wanted to have Phoebe hear the salvation message that he would preach under the anointing of the Holy Spirit. While attending the Theology Institute, I had learned that the anointing of the Holy Spirit is the painting or coming on of the Holy Spirit's presence over a person's life. Peter Youngren preached about Jesus feeding the five thousand men as well as the women and children present during lunchtime in the Bible days when Jesus walked the earth. I sensed a powerful anointing of the Holy Spirit in the church building that night, which was unusually stronger and people could sense.

I could hear Phoebe sniffling as Peter was preaching a powerful message that was touching her heart with the good news about the miracles of Jesus Christ.

When evangelist Peter Youngren had finished his preaching about the miracle of the multiplication of the fish and bread, he had given an invitation for those who would like to receive Jesus into their hearts and lives.

I thought about turning to Phoebe sitting on my right to see if she would like to accept Jesus into her heart, but I decided to leave it up to her and the Holy Spirit what she wanted to do at that moment.

To my surprise, Phoebe decided to raise her hand, signifying that she would like to receive Jesus into her heart that night. At Peter's invitation, Phoebe walked to the front of the church along with the other souls desirous to receive God's free gift of salvation through an act of inviting God into their lives in the person of Jesus Christ.

After saying the sinner's prayer after the evangelist, Phoebe and the others were led into a side room to be given further instructions on how to live for the Lord each day after accepting Christ Jesus.

When Phoebe came back out to where I was located in the congregation, a Christian man named Willard Houston, who also attended the church, came over to where Phoebe and I were. Willard shared with us that he had seen Phoebe before she accepted Christ Jesus in the church service, and he could see that her face had lit up after she accepted Jesus into her life. Phoebe was smiling with a big grin on her face, showing that she had received God's gift of salvation as is found in the person of Jesus Christ.

Phoebe shared with me after the service that when she heard that the disciples had turned their backs on the people who represented the need and they had looked to Jesus first, it really had touched her heart. Jesus met the spiritual needs of the people before he met their physical needs. Humanity worldwide has spiritual, emotional, mental, financial, social and family relationships, and physical needs that God in Christ is truly able to meet with abundance for those who truly place their faith and trust in the finished work of Jesus Christ on His cross which is resurrection validated. The Holy Spirit had brought home to her heart and life the wonderful truths of the miracle of Jesus as preached by Peter Youngren.

Before I drove Phoebe home, I decided to stop by a Christian senior citizen's home to have Phoebe tell the good news of receiving Jesus into her heart.

Once in the home of Charlene Spencer, my landlord, Phoebe walked up to Mrs. Spencer and gave her a big hug while saying to her, "I married Jesus."

I knew that something wonderful had happened in Phoebe's heart for a traditional religious person to say that she married Jesus. I kept in touch with Phoebe to see how she was doing in her new walk with Jesus in her life, and I recall how Phoebe shared with me over the phone that she had read in the Bible that Jesus had brothers and sisters. Phoebe was learning the wonderful truths about Jesus as revealed in the Bible for herself, and God the Holy Spirit was making the difference in her new life in Christ.

Phoebe had thought that she could serve the Lord by becoming a pious nun after she came to Christ. She was so sincere and precious in her new born-again, spiritual birth of a new nature in Christ Jesus, Christian walk with the living God that she was willing to serve the Lord any way she could think of. Phoebe stayed at a pious convent for nuns for three weeks. She later told me that she came to the realization that she could live for God without becoming a nun.

Phoebe wanted to find herself a good Christian church where she could grow in her new life in Christ. Phoebe told me that she decided not to attend the Evangel Christian Fellowship Church or the big Congregational Christian Church in Union. She also didn't want to make a Pentecostal Philippine Church in Union her church home. But when she found the Congregational Christian Church in Canton, Phoebe decided that it was the right Christian church, and she decided to make it her church home.

Phoebe had shared with me that when she was in the Philippines, she had gone to a Baptist church that emphasized the doctrine of water baptism as a required necessity for salvation; that was where she first heard the words of receiving Jesus into her heart. She remembered hearing those words at the Baptist church, but she hadn't responded to the invitation to receive Jesus at the time. After she accepted Jesus Christ into her heart at the Evangel Christian Fellowship Church, she continued to go to the Catholic Church, a traditional religious church, with her father in Union.

It was her father's wish that she remain in their traditional faith as observed and practiced culturally in the Philippines. She shared with me that she heard the priest say the words, "Receive Jesus into your heart," but it wasn't the same. Phoebe told me that she didn't feel she could grow in her new life in the traditional Catholic Church, and that was the reason that she began searching for the right Christian church, where she could grow in her new life in Christ Jesus.

I recognized that it was God the Holy Spirit at work in Phoebe's life, and He was doing a good work directing her steps before the Lord. I saw Phoebe at the Congregational Christian Church in Canton years later, and it was good to know that she had remained faithful to the Lord by her consistent attendance to the House of God over the years.

Phoebe is a living testimony that Jesus Christ can change a person's heart and life if that person will come to Him by faith for His free gift of salvation. It's important for the new believer in Christ to maintain a personal relationship with God through a faithful relationship with Jesus Christ, personal Lord and the Savior of his or her soul.

I learned a good lesson from watching Phoebe come to the Lord at the Evangel Christian Fellowship Church. I learned that whoever comes to know the Lord Jesus Christ, it can only happen through the power and operation of the Holy Spirit drawing that person to the Lord Jesus.

I had made the right choice of leaving the best work up to the Holy Spirit to work inside of Phoebe's heart and life, rather than for me wanting to move her toward salvation before the Lord had prepared her heart with His tender promptings when evangelist Peter Youngren had given the salvation invitation. I discovered that good things happen to them who wait on the Lord.

I remember thinking about the prospects of marrying Phoebe as a good Christian wife, but I balked at the idea when I thought about having children with her one day. I concluded that should we have children together, the children could turn out to be on the short size due to Phoebe—as well as her sweet parents—being short in stature. I recognized that Phoebe was a special lady with good qualities, but once again, I had certain qualities I was looking for in a wife, and being too short wasn't one of them. The Lord knew what qualities I was looking for in a wife, and I was willing to wait until I found that one special lady to marry.

I recall playing slow-pitch baseball for the Resurrection Life Church in Union. I found that I enjoyed pitching and playing right field on the Resurrection Life baseball team. One day when my team was having practice at Lake View Park, I happened to throw a ball in from the center field, which took one bounce and hit my teammate on the right buttocks. I called out to my Christian fellow member of the team to turn the other cheek. To that, I heard my teammates make a boo sound in unison to let me know that my remark wasn't considered to be the best thing to say coming from a Christian ballplayer. I found myself making the witty remark on the spur of the moment.

One day I had the opportunity to pitch against the Fairview Believer's Worship Center softball baseball team at Mountain View Park in Union. I had good control that day when I found myself pitching to a former professional football player named Mutu Swains.

When I was ahead on strikes, I liked to throw a high pitch that was considered above the strike zone before it made its descent right into the catcher's glove. Mutu waited on one of my high-pitched, out-of-the-strike-zone, throwaway pitches and knocked the ball completely out of the park. The ball sailed so high and long that it cleared the Mountain View Park fence and sailed into the tall trees, a long way past the silver wire home run fence.

I had given up five home runs to the big man in the two-game doubleheader when I saw him standing at home plate again for his turn at bat. I turned around to see if my coach, Jerry Alpha, wanted me to pitch to Mutu or gladly give him a free walk to first base. Jerry gave me the signal to go ahead and pitch to Mutu. Once again, the large Christian ballplayer taught me a lesson on how to hit a fat, juicy pitch out of the ballpark for home run number six. Thank goodness the big man is on the Lord's side, but it wasn't a pleasant day in the park for my teammates and me.

I surrendered two pitching losing games to Mutu and the Fairview Believer's Worship Center baseball team that day. I later discovered that Mutu Swains had played for the Seattle Seahawks before being traded to the San Francisco 49ers. He then played for the San Francisco 49ers as a defensive lineman.

I decided to join the William County Carrier summer baseball softball league, and I played for the Casaesar Carrier softball team for a couple of years in the nineties. I pitched every game that first year during our scheduled play for a carrier driver-player-coach Kent Martin. I recall the first year that I pitched for the Casaesar Carrier baseball team, the team won the regular season play with the most wins; but when it came time for tournament play at the end of the season, the team lost their opening game to the Rolland Carrier softball team at Lincoln Park in West Seattle.

We found ourselves put out of the tournament, disappointed with the crucial loss but determined to rally the baseball troops and play again the next softball season. The following year I once again found myself pitching every game on our game schedule. I found that I had excellent control when I threw my pitches with the back of my hand facing the home plate. When I released my pitches with my right arm extended high in the air, the softball tended to have plenty of backspin on the pitch. This seemed to create problems for the hitters, which gave me good success on the mound. I discovered that when I tried to pitch the soft ball with the palm of my hand facing home plate, I couldn't control my pitches.

The team's second softball season found my teammates and I losing our regular season play, but we won the tournament championship. When it came time for tournament play, my fellow ball club members and I found ourselves coming alive with consistent play at every position, intensity, and good power with the bats. My teammates and I were prolific with the bats in producing more runs than the opposing teams, and we won the William County softball tournament. When the team had a celebration get-together for our tournament victory later at the coach's home, I was honored by Kent Martin giving me an acknowledgement as the reason the team had won the championship. I appreciated hearing Kent's kind remark coming from the coach relative to being the leading cause for our success in winning the tournament play.

One late night, I decided to drop off several paper bags of leaves into the woods in the city I reside in south of Union. As a single man, I looked for ways to save money, and since I hadn't set up the extra yard waste service with my garbage account, I thought I could drop off the leaves into the woods and nobody would be the wiser. Driving down the steep street from my split-level home, I pulled over to park near the curb across from a secluded wooded area. There was a cement bulkhead on the north side of the street opposite my parked car that was an ideal area to empty the leaves over.

Wanting to be secretive and inconspicuous from any peering eyes, I dropped the contents of my yard waste over the side of the cement barrier. One of the sacks slipped out of my hands onto the ground below, and I started to think that the paper sack I dropped over the wall might have my fingerprints. I anxiously decided to retrieve the sack just in case someone found it and turned it in, revealing my sneaky save-some-bucks-in-the-cool-of-the-night actions. I had a nice long-sleeved jacket on that provided my arms some protection as I dropped over the side of the cement wall. Once I picked up the sack, now empty of the leaves, I discovered I wasn't tall enough to scale the wall to pull myself back up.

After repeated vain attempts of grabbing onto the flat top of the vertical tall barrier that prevented me from climbing back to my parked vehicle, I decided to put the leaves into a pile on the grass next to the wall. I hoped this would attain my goal of getting back to my car. I found that the piled-up bundle of leaves didn't help me to pull myself up onto the concrete wall. All of my efforts were futile in the cool of the dark night air. I was fortunate that no police came along to investigate my parked vehicle.

I was now faced with a real dilemma as to how I was going to get back home. There was the concrete wall I wasn't able to scale, and there were the blackberry vines along the tall barrier hindering my escape back up to freedom. I decided to work my way down the hillside through the tall, dense thicket to the street below, which ran along the side of a local park since I had on a long-sleeved jacket, blue jeans, and white tennis shoes. I soon found myself hung up by the dense thorny thicket protruding against my clothes, and I soon had to retrieve my tennis shoe that had gotten stuck in the soggy, muddy soil. I had thoughts of the fire department coming to my rescue to save me from the sticky clutches of the long-armed thorny thicket, with a camera crew filming the rescue only to be shown on the daily news.

I soon realized that I wasn't going to escape my predicament by working my way down the hillside of the compact, dense thicket of thorny overgrowth combined with the muddy ground. I slipped in the mud a number of times working my way back up to the side of the cement wall. In desperation, I decided to work my way along the side of the wall, with the short lip of ground coupled with blackberry vines protruding in a menacing manner hindering my progress, which slowed me down.

I was thinking of the time it was taking to escape my night ordeal in the woods. Looking back, I was grateful that I had the streetlights, which provided enough lighting for me to slowly make my way. Once again, I was finding that I wasn't going to walk out from my sticky captivity, with the blackberry vines forcing me to get to the point of realizing just how serious a predicament I was in. Finally I realized my way of escape from the blackberry vine captivity was to work my way back to the pile of leaves.

Painstakingly, I had to slowly work my way back to the stacked pile of leaves in front of the cement barrier that was restricting my escape to freedom each time I had attempted to climb up. I took more time to build up the pile of leaves into the tallest possible mound that I could make. I discovered that the extra time working on other ways to break free from my dark predicament had allowed me to recover the energy level necessary to pull myself up from the dangers I was facing. My jacket experienced scrape marks from my brush with the concrete wall, but I was finally free.

My newfound freedom was a real reward for my abilities to persevere in the face of difficult circumstances. I had anxiously kept myself busy, partly out of fear of being found by a police officer wondering exactly why I had abandoned my vehicle in the first place and what I was doing in the woods late at night. The dark skies and the environment would have caused suspicion.

When I drove back home, I called my girlfriend, Bobbie Jo, to tell her about the predicament I had just gotten through experiencing in the woods. While I was talking to Bobbie Jo, worn out from my harrowing experience, I heard a loud, piercing scream from the cat that I was taking care of for a friend. The male gray and white tiger-striped cat was named

Sneakers because all of his feet were white as if he had white tennis shoes on. Sneakers had a powerful dislike for my female cat named Fluffy. I was keeping Sneakers in the spare bedroom upstairs away from my two female cats. All the cats had been fixed to help reduce the pet population. Somehow when I was out on my night outing, Sneakers had escaped from the small bedroom where he had been enclosed with the door firmly shut.

Hearing the loud, piercing scream through my open bedroom door, I immediately jumped up from lying on my bed to quickly come to the rescue of my gray, long-haired cat Fluffy.

I knew from the angry mountain lion screams that Sneakers had Fluffy trapped, and I grabbed a plastic hanger to scare Sneakers away from tearing into my mild-mannered pet. I turned on the light in the short hallway offset from my basement bedroom and headed directly toward the loud, angry screams. I was able to see Sneakers in the dim light just inside of the partially open door of the entertainment room.

I took two swipes with the plastic hanger at Sneakers, at which point, Sneakers leaped up, grabbing with his claws into my descending right arm. The sudden, painful attack had surprised me. I was in shock that Sneakers would make a bold move to attack me as violently as a fierce tomcat. I was able to free myself from the clinging creature and get Sneakers to retreat back up the stairs of my split-level house.

When I looked at my right arm, I saw the bloody wounds from where I was attacked by the angry tomcat filled with rage toward the mild-mannered Fluffy.

After saving Fluffy from Sneakers, I contacted Bobbie Jo at her apartment in Collard. As I told her of the painful attack by the savage tomcat, Bobbie Jo was thinking that I might need to go to the Fairmont Medical Center in Collard for a tetanus shot.

I listened to what Bobbie Jo had to say, but I declined to have her drive me or drive myself to the hospital so early in the morning; it was still dark outside. I concluded that Sneaker's care at the Scone residence was now over; I recognized that the tomcat needed a home where he could be cared for by a nice senior citizen without any other cats representing competition for attention. I was able to get Sneakers back into his bedroom enclosure with the aid of a good, trusty broom, and that put an end to my night of terror and scary encounters.

I was soon able to talk with Jake Williams, who assured me that he knew of a woman who would provide a good home for Sneakers. Jake had done a lot of yard work for me, so I trusted that Jake was on the level and Sneakers would have a caring home where he could be the king of his own domain. Later, when I checked with Jake about Sneakers to find out how he was, Jake let me know that once I give a pet away, I shouldn't inquire about the pet.

I was surprised by Jake's response to a simple question, and I later concluded that Jake had disposed of the cat, even though I couldn't prove it one way or the other. I had at least tried to find another caring home for Sneakers by entrusting the care of the cat into Jake's custody to find a good home for the ferocious feline, although Sneakers had taught me a lesson about the unpredictability of domestic animals, which may turn wild when they encounter another animal of like kind.

One day as I was listening to the radio while driving my car, I heard an advertisement about a cosmetic surgeon practicing at the Open Door Surgery Center in Champus. I called the phone number that was given over the radio and made an appointment to see Lowell Piper, MD, who did facial plastic surgeries. I also went to see Alfred Thompson, MD, a double-board plastic surgeon in Union. "Double-board" means certified in two specialties: general surgery and plastic ophthalmology and plastic ent and plastic reconstruction surgery," according to a certified American Board Plastic Surgeon, Dr. R. R.

I learned that Dr. Piper wanted twenty-nine hundred for a rhinoplasty-nose job, and Dr. Thompson wanted five thousand for the same cosmetic surgery procedure. I came to the no-brainer conclusion, which was to go for the less expensive one.

In the nineties, I had my first rhinoplasty cosmetic surgery with Dr. Piper for a sum total of thirty-one hundred dollars, including tax. I found that I wasn't satisfied with my nose surgery results, and at a later date in the nineties, I had my second rhinoplasty with Dr. James Evans, a double-board plastic surgeon, to reduce the bridge of my nose some more, evenly balance the nostrils, and reduce the tip of the nose a little bit more if at all possible.

I didn't like the postsurgery results initially, but in time, when my nose had softened and relaxed postsurgery, I found that I liked the doctor's cosmetic work. Later, I did become self-conscious about my left nostril being somewhat higher elevated than my right nostril due to missing cartilage. This made me self-conscious about people who would talk to me on my left side, as opposed to those standing on my right side who wanted to talk with me.

I had my ears and chin worked on by a plastic surgeon named Christopher Smith, MD, also in the nineties. I remember being under a local anesthesia and being able to feel the pain as Dr. Smith was cutting on my ears. I also remember how persistent Dr. Smith was in hitting on the African American nursing assistant in the surgery room to get together with her at a later time.

I discovered some time later that Dr. Smith was nearing the end of his career as a plastic surgeon, and I believe now that Smith was interested in adding me to his professional statistics. I discovered that I wasn't pleased with my cosmetic results postsurgery, and I inquired if Dr. Smith could perform a second surgery on my right ear to try to get the contour evenly balanced with the left ear. I found that the second surgery on my right ear wasn't a positive success either.

I now wish I had not had any surgeries on my ears because they were fine to begin with. I had been thinking at the time of my initial surgeries that I would like to have my ears brought in somewhat to have a good-looking natural shape, as I saw actors on television have. It's obvious to me that, like so many other would-be cosmetic consumers, I was influenced by physical beauty glamorized in Hollywood pictures and portrayed on television and in the movies.

I recognize that I can't blame Hollywood for my poor cosmetic results, but I realize that I was influenced to pursue having cosmetic surgeries because physical beauty is recognized as the in-thing to seek after to be accepted by other beautiful people. I have come to recognize that the world has a lot of fool's gold that people are seeking after that will leave them feeling empty, used, and abused by profiteers and exploiters in this world's system if they are not careful.

I have appreciated the different quips and quotes that my mother, Jessica, would say at times. One quote she learned from her cousin Ralph Jorganson, who used to live in Spokane before he passed away. It was the

The Ultimate Violation

following: "I know how handsome I are, I know that my face is no star. But my face, I don't mind it. It's the folks in front that gets the jar."

I have come to realize that any potential surgical patient and cosmetic consumer needs to ask a lot of questions regarding the medical doctor before he or she ever proceeds to have cosmetic surgery in the first place. I was able to acquire a couple of excellent questions to ask a cosmetic or plastic surgeon from a female staff member who took my phone call; plastic surgeons happen to work at the medical center she works at. The two questions are: "Who are you board certified through?" And "What are your qualifications?"

I encourage the reader to ask for names and phone numbers of satisfied customers from the doctor or from his office staff to get a good idea of what you may expect when it comes to postsurgery results.

Be specific as much as you want to be concerning the cosmetic procedure and postsurgery results because when it comes to your face, you want to have the right, qualified cosmetic or plastic surgeon work on your facial features.

I was informed before surgery that Dr. Lowell Piper, who did my first rhinoplasty, was an ENT. Dr. Piper was specialized in the ear, nose, and throat, and that gave me confidence to go with him initially.

I recognize now that I would have preferred to have my nose work done by Dr. Alfred Thompson, who is a certified double-board plastic surgeon in Union. I wish I had paid the five thousand dollars for the extra-qualified plastic surgeon in the first place, rather than go for extra surgeries to have my nose work corrected at a later time by a plastic surgeon. I have come to realize the importance of finding the right plastic or cosmetic surgeon for a consumer from the start, rather than continuing to go for additional surgeries to reach the right cosmetic look.

I wish that Dr. Piper had referred me to Dr. Thompson, who had the additional certified qualifications that I now see would have been important to have for my nose procedure.

I caution the reader to do your homework before you decide to make an appointment with the medical doctor who you want to do the cosmetic procedure on whatever body part you're desiring physical beauty enhancements for. Your future happiness depends on finding the right plastic surgeon for you. It is very important for your mental health that, postsurgery, you are confident you did find the right cosmetic surgeon for yourself and you can move forward in life with a bright future feeling successful. You never want to live with regret, as I have had to throughout the years. I now realize I wasn't properly educated or informed and I did not have a good understanding of what I could expect with each of my pre- and postsurgery cosmetic procedures and results. I have come to realize that cosmetic surgery can be a scary proposition in the wrong surgeon's hands.

I know from firsthand experience that there are cosmetic surgeons who are willing to use and exploit you as a guinea pig for their own self-interests, professional gain, and personal profits. I want the reader to move forward toward cosmetic surgery only after being properly educated and well informed with each step that he or she might take that results in cosmetic or plastic surgery.

THE ENCOUNTER

I recall looking in the yellow pages at an advertisement of how to find the right cosmetic or plastic surgeon for yourself. I had patiently waited for nearly five years, and I was interested in seeing if there was anything that a plastic or cosmetic surgeon might be able to surgically do to bring down my left nostril to be equal with the right nostril. I had been self-conscious when I was with family, friends, and acquaintances long enough, and I felt that if anything could be done to correct the imbalance of the nostrils on my nose, it was worth having it surgically corrected by a qualified medical surgeon.

I had completely forgotten the woman who used to work for Dr. Alfred Thompson, who is a double-board plastic surgeon in Union. The candid assistant had informed me that if you want to have nose surgery, you want to have it done by a double-board plastic surgeon.

When I saw the full-page ad for Thadeaus Damon Cutter, MD, in the yellow pages, I had completely forgotten all about the excellent advice offered to me by Dr. Thompson's assistant back in the nineties. I had concluded from seeing Dr. Cutter's full-page ad that if he couldn't do cosmetically what I was interested in, the doctor would refer me to another doctor who could do what I wanted and needed.

When I made my phone call to Dr. Cutter's cosmetic office in Union, I informed the receptionist, named Alice, that I had two previous nose surgeries. Alice told me that Dr. Cutter frequently has patients who come to him that have had previous surgeries with other doctors.

I asked about the ad I'd seen in the yellow pages (from another doctor) on how to find the right beauty enhancement or physical characteristics surgeon for yourself. I told Alice that I was seeing listings for both plastic and cosmetic surgeons in the yellow pages, and I inquired the difference between the two. Alice told me that they are basically the same. Upon hearing her short response, I made my appointment with Dr. Cutter.

When I went to Dr. Cutter's office, I met with Dr. Cutter's photo technician and nursing assistant before I met with the cosmetic surgeon himself. I recall the woman acting a little nervous, but at the time, I didn't question her demeanor beyond the surface. She told me that if she could have cosmetic surgery on her nose over again, she would have Dr. Cutter perform the surgery. I understood her comment as satisfaction with her first-time rhinoplasty procedure and that she would not proceed with a second rhinoplasty procedure even if she could afford it. Dr. Cutter's photo technician never stated that she was waiting to have Dr. Cutter surgically perform another rhinoplasty on her nose, and that it was only a matter of coming up with the money to pay for the cost of surgery that had delayed the scheduled date for her second rhinoplasty procedure. She was only making a statement, which I now recognize was her way of building up my confidence to proceed with having my third rhinoplasty with Dr. Cutter because of how good he was with noses. The assistant took a number of photos of my face, and then I waited for my opportunity to meet with Dr. Cutter.

I recall that when I met with Dr. Cutter, my first statement was, "I'd like to see if my left nostril could be brought down to be equal with the right."

I recall that Dr. Cutter didn't say anything as he stood up, turned around, and faced the wall.

When Dr. Cutter was silent facing the wall, I broke the silence with, "It must be hard to bring it down once it's up."

With those words spoken by me, Dr. Cutter turned back around and proceeded to sit down across from me. Dr. Cutter went on to say a couple of nonpertinent things that didn't address my cosmetic concerns.

Dr. Cutter then looked right at me and said, "I see ten different things wrong with your nose."

When I heard Dr. Cutter address my nose in such a way, it caused me to think I had found the right cosmetic surgeon for myself. I had my hopes built up by the women who worked for Dr. Cutter as assistants, who informed me that he was good with noses, and by the words communicated by Dr. Cutter. Dr. Cutter had a team of women working for him, including the receptionist, the nursing assistant (who was the photo technician), and even the blond-haired woman who had spoken with me before I filled out all the credit card information to pay for my surgeries. Each one had a role to play in building up my confidence on how good the medical doctor was with noses. Postsurgery, I realize that

Dr. Cutter's staff of female employees positively had a direct influence on my thinking that I could expect beauty enhancements for my nose.

Dr. Cutter then moved me to his computer imagery room, where my left side profile was clearly visible on his computer monitor. With a click on his computer mouse, Dr. Cutter said, "How about this?"

The monitor screen revealed my nose having a subtle change, with a straight bridge and a minimal reduction to the tip of my nose.

The corrections Dr. Cutter was clearly advertising to his cosmetic inquirer were to be corrected in the exact same position he had found my nose, as clearly shown on his computer monitor screen. Dr. Cutter never suggested in the slightest way to me that he might need to elevate my nose in order to achieve his goal of straightening my banana-shaped nose, as he referred to it. I was mentally focused on what Dr. Cutter was advertising to his potential patient precisely because of what my nose would look like postsurgery. I never imagined at this juncture that Dr. Cutter had plans of raising and repositioning my nose, which became the abject horror that I experienced postsurgery. I have learned that nonrecognized medical board doctors will utilize computer imagery to capture the attention of a potential patient, but the cosmetic results may be painfully contrary to the beauty enhancement imagery portrayed on the doctor's computer monitor.

When I saw the subtle change to my nose on the computer monitor, which I found appealing, I found myself saying, "Yeah!"

After all, Dr. Cutter wasn't advertising a major change that would cause me something to be concerned about at a later date.

In hindsight, I know that Dr. Cutter did not tell me of his status of not being certified by any one of the twenty-four boards of medical specialties. Dr. Cutter and his assistants were leading me to believe that he was a specialist in the nose and ears. I have come to recognize that Dr. Cutter has a "Don't ask, don't tell" cosmetic status policy.

Just to make absolutely certain I hadn't missed something from his full-page cosmetic ad in the yellow pages, I would have appreciated Dr. Cutter communicating that he was not a board-certified plastic surgeon or a reconstruction cosmetic surgeon.

Should I possibly not understand his Outpatient Board Certification medical status, his American Board of Oral Maxiallofacial Surgery status, and his nonrecognized American Board of Cosmetic Surgery status, I know Dr. Cutter should have informed me exactly how these medical trainings had prepared him to start doing additional cutting on my nose and ears above and beyond what Dr. Piper, Dr. Evans, and Dr. Smith had surgically done. Had Dr. Cutter been more forthright in his communication with me, I might have had a little more respect for him than I did postsurgery.

Dr. Cutter's storming-the-brain tactics included a blitzkrieg of new information as a sudden attack to the brain by catching the patient mentally off guard so that the patient begins to think and question in his or her mind why the doctor hadn't explained his plans before the day of surgery, and then a quick application of hypnotic paralysis to the mind, where the subdued patient has then no options to consider on the day of surgery. These tactics were not appreciated by me postsurgery. Dr. Cutter had appeared to provide me with options during my initial consultation and my second consultation, but positively he made certain for his subdued patient there were no other options but to have the surgeries with his surgical instruments as hastily as possible after receiving anesthesia. I had explained everything to Dr. Cutter in my postsurgery desired results notes, a copy of which Dr. Cutter had requested, but Dr. Cutter had totally omitted discussing whether he could or couldn't fulfill my specifications concerning my cosmetic interests and postsurgery expectations.

This was not understood initially postsurgery. The long and slow process that I had to painfully endure gradually allowed me to come to a full realization years later exactly what Dr. Cutter had done to me pre- and postsurgery.

Dr. Cutter took me into a separate room, where I found myself inquiring if he could correct the bent curve in my nose. Dr. Cutter thought he could do that. I don't know if my nose had a natural bent to it when I was born or whether the bridge of my nose happened to get slightly bent when I had a collision with a catcher at home plate during a baseball game when I was a teenager.

I recall telling Dr. Cutter that my first rhinoplasty was with Dr. Piper.

Dr. Cutter responded by saying, "He's an ENT," referring to an ear, nose, and throat cosmetic surgeon.

I shared with Dr. Cutter that I had my second rhinoplasty with Dr. Evans. Dr. Cutter said, "He's a plastic surgeon."

At one point during the second consultation, Dr. Cutter told me that my nose and chin would be easy, but my ears would be tricky because they might relapse back inward once he tried to bring them out away from my head.

I found myself thinking that I was willing to have this surgical procedure done in order to evenly balance my ears away from the side of my head, resolving the imbalance created by Dr. Smith's two separate ottoplasty surgical procedures on my right ear, and one ottoplasty surgery procedure on my left ear, as a consequence of the ear surgeries I had years previously.

I thought I was dealing with a specialist in the nose and ears at this point, and not a cosmetic con artist trying to deceive, dupe, and scam an unsuspecting patient with cosmetic fantasy words and images dangled before a cosmetic hopeful.

I left Dr. Cutter's cosmetic practice that day thinking I had finally found the right surgeon, who could correct my physical characteristics with good-quality results.

I remember talking to my coworker Denise after the initial consultation about thinking I had found the right cosmetic surgeon for myself. Denise inquired of me whether Dr. Cutter had a qualified anesthesiologist. My response to Denise was, "I'm sure he does."

I was assuming that Dr. Cutter had a professional practice in proper order and that any concern that Denise might have about his practice was surely accounted for with qualified assistants who worked for him. When I came back in to see Dr. Cutter for our second consultation, I was going to make certain he could cosmetically do what I wanted and needed. I took the time to write out specific postsurgery desired results notes; I wanted Dr. Cutter to tell me whether he could cosmetically do what I was interested in.

I recall Dr. Cutter holding a photo album open several feet away from me and telling me about a male patient that he had performed surgery on. Dr. Cutter never handed the photo album to me for me to examine the cosmetic results for myself. In retrospect, I can see how Dr. Cutter set me up to perform cosmetic surgeries on my nose, ears, and chin. It was something that I would come to regret for years and years spent in agonizing mental and emotional pain, humiliation, self-consciousness, and shame.

When I showed Dr. Cutter my handwritten notes during our second consultation, Dr. Cutter held the notes in his hands and said, "I want to make a copy for myself." Dr. Cutter then said, "This gives me something to work with."

As Dr. Cutter started to walk away, he stopped halfway to the doorway, turned around, and while looking at me, he said, "I'm a perfectionist." Dr. Cutter then turned and walked out of the room.

When Dr. Cutter came back into the consultation room where I was patiently waiting, he gave me my notes back. I recognize that Dr. Cutter and I never went over my postsurgery desired results notes regarding whether Dr. Cutter could cosmetically do what I wanted and needed.

I now see that Dr. Cutter wasn't saying a lot of things. I now know for a fact that Dr. Cutter should have done a lot more communicating with me from the patient's perspective—especially since Dr. Cutter knew what his next move was going to be cosmetically, without me knowing what he was going to cosmetically do. Had Dr. Cutter communicated more during our initial consultation, he would have lost my cosmetic and financial business, but he would have gained my respect.

I came to realize postsurgery that Dr. Cutter only wanted my cosmetic and financial business, so he kept his communication with me to a minimum. When I reflect back upon my encounter with Dr. Cutter, I recognize that Dr. Cutter was adept at keeping me mentally off balance and mentally starved for more detailed information.

I left Dr. Cutter's cosmetic practice that day trusting that Dr. Cutter knew what I wanted and needed cosmetically.

I came to realize that my approaching surgery date was on Dr. Cutter's schedule, but I still needed some additional assurance that the medical doctor knew exactly what I was desiring and hoping for postsurgery. Since I was going to have the three surgeries for my nose, ears, and chin on the same day, instead of paying twelve thousand dollars, I would get a discount and only have to pay eleven thousand four hundred dollars. I was pleased to know that I was going to get a financial discount on my cosmetic surgeries toward my physical enhancements.

I was looking forward to the new look with anticipation, and I had something important to show Dr. Cutter. I decided to bring in a videotape of *The Accidental Tourist* starring the actor William Hurt to let Dr. Cutter take a look at the actor's nose.

I had a male passenger who rode one of my William County Carrier shuttle routes comment that I looked like William Hurt. I accepted the comment by the male passenger as a compliment because I considered the actor to be a handsome man with a good-looking nose.

When I wanted Dr. Cutter to view the videotape where he could visually see the actor's nose for himself, Dr. Cutter commented that he didn't want to see the video because he knew the actor. I recall that I was really disappointed that Dr. Cutter didn't want to take any time to observe the physical appearance of the actor's nose because I was interested in having my nose look like that actor's nose.

I recall becoming perplexed and feeling disappointed that Dr. Cutter did not want to take the time to see even a small portion of the video I brought in on the day of my surgeries. Dr. Cutter was looking down at his hands on the table in the consultation room. I recall that I was feeling mentally perplexed and disappointed over the situation that he had left a lot unmentioned, when Dr. Cutter stood up and moved directly behind me. He then said, "Well, I better go about building up the bridge."

As I thought upon Dr. Cutter's words, I wondered why he hadn't told this to me before the day of surgery. As I followed Dr. Cutter into the next room, which was darkened, my mind went suddenly blank from the hypnotic whammy Dr. Cutter had assaulted me with. I didn't know what hit me until years later when I eventually figured out in my mind precisely how I had become a patient of Dr. Cutter's. I remember questioning in my mind why Dr. Cutter hadn't told me up front of his plans to build up the bridge of my nose, which was not at all in my notes of which Dr. Cutter had wanted a copy for himself. I eventually came to realize Dr. Cutter's hypnotic whammy that the medical doctor had utilized on me preceded receiving anesthesia for my surgeries.

I remember waking up from surgery while I was still on the surgery table and hearing Dr. Cutter say, "You're going to like it."

I was mentally dull after surgery when my coworker Denise Montgomery provided a ride home for me.

Ten days postsurgery, I came back in to have my stitches removed at Dr. Cutter's cosmetic practice. I remember having Dr. Cutter's assistant explain to me that he was in the surgery room on the day of my surgeries. After I had two sutures removed from my nostrils and my stitches taken out from my nose, Dr. Cutter's assistant left the room.

As I was sitting down with my legs resting on Dr. Cutter's dental chair, I recall Dr. Cutter entering the room and standing next to me. Dr. Cutter said to me, "See it as a sculpture. I tore it down, beat it up, and built it back up." He then left the room.

Upon hearing the words communicated to me by Dr. Cutter, I began reflecting how his words articulated in detail his cosmetic actions during my surgeries. I found myself reflecting over and over again on Dr. Cutter's words spoken to me relative to seeing it as a sculpture; having it torn down and built back up seemed to be a total disconnect between the cosmetic surgeon and the patient. I came to recognize that something had gone horribly wrong with our communication, and I wondered why the medical doctor hadn't told me the total truth of his plans and what he had envisioned before my surgeries. I came to recognize that I couldn't believe that a medical doctor would ever tell a sensitive multisurgery patient such bizarre things, which seemed totally insensitive and callous. I came to the mentally agonizing realization that I had encountered the wrong medical doctor for my cosmetic needs as I reflected on his words and the contrary results I experienced. I began to question in my mind *If that's what he had envisioned doing, why didn't he tell me that up front during our initial consultation?*

The more I reflected upon Dr. Cutter's words spoken to me postsurgery, the more they began to bother me. I found myself continuously searching in my mind and racking my brain, perplexed by what Dr. Cutter had done to me cosmetically.

I wondered: *Why did this happen to me? And how could something as horrifying as this cosmetic nightmare have happened to me? Why did Dr. Cutter say the kind of things he had spoken to me after my surgeries, and clearly not before my surgeries?*

I found myself constantly thinking, reflecting, . rehashing, and rethinking again and again how I had encountered Dr. Cutter, a medical doctor who did completely opposite what I wanted, needed, and expected for my nose and ears.

My cosmetic experience was devastatingly painful and mentally confusing to say the least. What kind of a doctor would wait until after surgery to tell me, "See it as a sculpture. I tore it down, beat it up, and built it back up?" Postsurgery I found myself looking at the cosmetic changes to my facial features in the mirror, uncertain of the real detailed changes at first. I also would videotape myself so I could observe the changes made to my nose, ears, and chin on my large-screen TV, rather than relying on the smaller images of myself in the viewfinder on my camcorder. I would closely examine, scrutinize, and inspect Dr. Cutter's cosmetic work on my facial features over and over for long periods of time. I had begun to carefully examine the changes that Dr. Cutter had made to my facial features after the adhesive-taped plastic molding had fallen off of my nose while I was taking a shower one day. I began trying to determine if the changes I could clearly see as reflected in the mirror or as played back for my viewing on the TV were physically positive for an improved new look for myself or were the changes positively not for the better, but a detriment toward my overall physical appearance.

Within the first couple of months following my surgeries, I found the cosmetic changes were diametrically opposite of what I wanted, needed, and expected. I began to experience the painful mental and emotional agony, and the commencing of the incredible suffering I would undergo, as the painful results from my postsurgeries, which were now causing me to experience a nasty case of deep mental and emotional depression. The postsurgery results eventually became so horribly revealing that they showed my nose had been physically elevated, raised, and repositioned, giving me the impression of it looking like a turtle-shaped nose. My ears initially appeared to have been brought out away from the side of my head, and within a matter of weeks, they had relapsed back in now closer than my presurgery position in relation to the side of my head. When it came to my chin, the skin pigment tissues had changed color from a flesh tone to a reddish color tone, which became the cause of why I wanted to grow my beard once again to cover up the embarrassment of my discolored chin with reddish skin pigment.

I became painfully aware that I had chosen the wrong medical doctor for my personal cosmetic needs, and with time I came to the conclusion that these cosmetic crimes should have never taken place. Had the right policies of the medical board been honorably upheld, enforced, and exclusively restrictive so that only board-certified plastic surgeons recognized by the twenty-four boards of medical specialties, the ABMS, would be allowed to perform cosmetic or reconstruction surgical procedures on multiple-surgery patients, I would never have had any surgeries with Dr. Thadeaus Damon Cutter.

I am an advocate for completely putting a stop to and preventing medical malpractice by medical doctors and medical negligence caused by professional personnel in hospitals throughout the country.

I believe it can be done provided the legal and medical authorities wake up to the physical atrocities taking place against innocent patients throughout Victimized, USA. It's high time the laws and policies supposedly being upheld by the health commissions in each state of the union recognize that there are predators disguised as caring medical doctors among their board memberships.

I recognize that my book is timely regarding this serious subject matter, and it's time for every medical commission in this great country to see what is happening under their questionable caring eyes.

I found myself examining my physical appearance by repeatedly looking in the mirror and examining my appearance with my video camera postsurgery. The more I examined the facial features of my new look and how my appearance wasn't what I expected it to be, I found myself becoming increasingly unhappy with Dr. Cutter's cosmetic results. Each day following my cosmetic surgeries caused me to reflect continuously upon Dr. Cutter and the actions that he had taken against me on the day of surgery.

When I saw my reflection in the handheld mirror and in the various mirrors throughout my home south of Union, I became increasingly saddened by what I saw.

I decided to make an appointment with Craig Cranberry, MD, to get his professional opinion regarding Dr. Cutter's cosmetic results. I had made an appointment with Dr. Cranberry before having my surgeries with Dr. Cutter, and I was interested in hearing what Dr. Cranberry had to say concerning my postsurgery results.

During my appointment, Dr. Cranberry commented that he thought my nose was better than what I had before surgery. I was surprised by Dr. Cranberry's remark that my nose looked better now than before. I found out sometime postsurgery that Dr. Cranberry was a friend of Dr. Cutter's. Dr. Cranberry had told me during our consultation that he was not a plastic surgeon, but that he had worked with a plastic surgeon before. I remember looking through some photo albums of Dr. Cranberry's work, and I thought from the postsurgery pictures that he did good-quality work.

I left Dr. Cranberry's office not satisfied with what I had heard regarding my postsurgery results. I decided to get a second opinion from another cosmetic surgeon whom I had seen prior to having surgeries with Dr. Cutter.

I made an appointment to see Chris Kirtpatrick, MD, to get his professional opinion regarding Dr. Cutter's postsurgery cosmetic results. Dr. Kirtpatrick had told me that he was a triple-board cosmetic surgeon, and I thought that Dr. Kirtpatrick understood my cosmetic interests when I had communicated exactly what I was wanting him to cosmetically do. Dr. Kirtpatrick had understood that I wanted to have my left nostril brought back down to be evenly matched and balanced with my right side nostril. I wasn't interested in having the bridge of my nose built up nor the tip of my nose raised in order to correct the imbalance with my nostrils, so I never mentioned the two separate aspects to Dr. Kirtpatrick. When I heard Dr. Kirtpatrick mention during our initial consultation that he would build up the bridge and raise the tip of my nose, I decided not to have nose surgery with Dr. Kirtpatrick. I decided to continue my search for the right cosmetic or plastic surgeon for myself after leaving Dr. Kirtpatrick's cosmetic office that day.

Now I was coming in to see Dr. Kirtpatrick for his professional evaluation regarding Dr. Cutter's cosmetic work. Dr. Kirtpatrick took a look at the notes that Dr. Cutter had told me gave him something to work with, which he had copied for himself.

After Dr. Kirtpatrick looked at my postsurgery desired results notes, he said, "There must have been a misunderstanding." I had mentioned to Dr. Kirtpatrick that I was thinking of suing Dr. Cutter, which I later concluded I shouldn't have mentioned to the medical doctor because it might get back to Dr. Cutter. Dr. Kirtpatrick wanted to know if I wanted him to act as a mediator between me and Dr. Cutter.

As a consequence, I agreed to sign a consent form for Dr. Kirtpatrick to perform and fulfill his mediatory position between me and Dr. Cutter. I had initially thought that Dr. Cutter had taken my nose in the wrong direction of what I was wanting and needing cosmetically. Now was a good time to hear what other doctors had to say of Dr. Cutter's cosmetic results.

I had made my appointments to see Dr. Cranberry and Dr. Kirtpatrick before coming back in to see Dr. Cutter approximately three months after my surgeries. I recall that once again, Dr. Cutter's nursing and photo assistant had taken pictures of my postsurgeries' new cosmetic look. I and my coworker Denise—I had wanted a witness when I talked to Dr. Cutter regarding the cosmetic changes he had made primarily to my nose—had waited patiently to see Dr. Cutter, and he eventually came into the computer imagery room and sat down next to me.

I pointed out how my left side nostril had been raised during my surgeries, and Dr. Cutter cut me off by saying, "You are this close to terminating the doctor-patient relationship." Dr. Cutter went on to say, "You went to see a couple of my colleagues without my permission."

Dr. Cutter communicated that I had done something unethical by seeing his colleagues without getting his permission. Dr. Cutter said, "I have a lot of critics. Do you want their phone numbers?"

I said no to Dr. Cutter's direct question. I found myself completely caught off guard by Dr. Cutter's in-your-face response, and I was still mentally dull in light of wanting to have Dr. Cutter explain to me what he had cosmetically done to my nose.

Dr. Cutter then stood up, walked over in front of the doorway, and said while looking right at me, "You can sue me. You can blackmail me. I don't care what you do—you're not getting your money back."

When I heard Dr. Cutter's statement regarding not getting my money back, I spoke up and said, "I'd like my money back."

When Denise saw the way Dr. Cutter was not acting like a professional doctor, she interjected by saying to Dr. Cutter, "He has difficulty going out into public places." I appreciated having my coworker Denise speak up to Dr. Cutter on my behalf, and I felt that her remark was accurate, succinctly stated, and most appropriate to say to the medical doctor on the attack. I had been totally devastated by the cosmetic results caused by Dr Cutter's nonrecognized board certification surgical procedures on my facial features. The ABMS, the American Board of Medical Specialties, and ABPS, the American Board of Plastic Surgery, do not recognize the board certification given to Dr. Cutter. I absolutely had extremely painful difficulties going out into the public arena, where the general public could look at my abnormal facial disfigurement caused by Dr. Cutter's actions forged upon my facial features.

Dr. Cutter responded to Denise while he stared right at me, "Well, if I knew he had mental problems, I never would have done it."

Denise shared with Dr. Cutter that I videotaped myself with my camcorder. To that, Dr. Cutter responded by saying, "He needs to throw his camcorder away."

I recall that Dr. Cutter stood momentarily by me, moved over to one side of the room, and, looking up, said, "Noooooo!"

I didn't know what Dr. Cutter was doing at the time, but I now believe that Dr. Cutter had a sudden revelation that what he had done to me was a big mistake on his part. I am convinced that at that moment, Dr. Cutter knew he had hurt an innocent, unsuspecting patient, but he also knew that he couldn't retract his cosmetic tyranny against me.

Dr. Cutter took me into a separate room, which I now believe was his dimly lit, presurgery room where he performed his psychological whammy on me. He said to me, "Didn't I show you a right side profile of your nose and what I was going to do?"

Dr. Cutter acted totally surprised when he heard me respond boldly to his question, "No, you didn't." I went on to try and explain that Dr. Cutter had shown me a left side profile of my nose, and with a click of his computer mouse, he said, "How about this?" I found myself reaching a point where I began fumbling over my words, and I came to a stop. I found that it was not worth continuing to explain what had happened next.

I remember saying to Dr. Cutter that I had gone to see Dr. Thompson, who told me that he was double-board certified. I went on to tell Dr. Cutter that I had seen Dr. Kirtpatrick, who told me he is triple-board certified. I said, "I never let them touch my nose." I added, "I don't even know what your qualifications are."

When I finished saying, "I don't even know what your qualifications are," Dr. Cutter became silent on the subject. Dr. Cutter *never* explained to me what his qualifications were to be doing additional cosmetic work on a multiple-surgery patient.

Before I left my postsurgery consultation with Dr. Cutter, I looked up directly into his face and said, "I do not like it."

Dr. Cutter told me that I had ruined his night because he had a meeting to go to. It wasn't Dr. Cutter's facial characteristics that had been violated by me performing cosmetic surgical procedures on Dr. Cutter, but Dr. Cutter had gone to extreme lengths to prove that he wasn't the skilled plastic surgeon that I was wanting and needing for my cosmetic interests. Dr. Cutter forged ahead utilizing hypnotic assault tactics against my free-thinking associations in my mind for me to consider my options of having surgery or not having surgery, in order to subdue his patient so that I was unable to respond in a normal manner. I came to recognize him as going to extreme lengths and drastic measures to plunder and apprehend my financial and cosmetic business.

The above postsurgery realizations were gradually recognized by me because of what Dr. Cutter had done to my mind. I came to realize that it took a full eight to nine years of meditating and cogitating over and over in my mind on my dark encounter with Dr. Cutter on the day of my surgeries, until I finally worked it through and broke free of the mental restraints in my thoughts to completely figure out and envision what happened to me as I followed Dr. Cutter into a dark room. I experienced sudden mental blankness in his presurgery dimly lit room under his hypnotic mental manipulation tactics.

Postsurgery, Dr. Cutter's hypnotic assault on me was like having a strong mental straitjacket placed on my mind to prevent and restrain me from thinking clearly and freely. It kept me from figuring out exactly what Dr. Cutter had done to me mentally, and how he had been able to apprehend my financial and cosmetic business in the first place. I came to realize Dr. Cutter's actions were a total waste of my mental, emotional, spiritual, and physical being; they became utter torment inflicted on an innocent, unsuspecting patient. Postsurgery, I came to realize that as a multisurgery patient with everything I had experienced and suffered caused by the mental manipulation and surgical actions of Dr. Cutter, that I was violated and victimized by a sadistic medical predator.

Dr. Cutter was *braggadocio* in his haughty arrogance to me and showed that he was the master of my cosmetic destiny when he triumphantly said, "See it as a sculpture. I tore it down, beat it up, and built it back up."

I did not ask Dr. Cutter to tear down the previous doctor's cosmetic and plastic surgical work during our consultations together, nor was that work stated in my postsurgery desired results notes.

Dr. Cutter had misinterpreted just who I am as a person. I clearly was not a man for Dr. Cutter to take malicious cosmetic liberties with my physical characteristics when Dr. Cutter was not a specialist in the nose and ears.

Dr. Cutter thought he could get away with his cosmetic violations, butcheries, and deviations and I was supposed to sit idly by and do absolutely nothing about it. I didn't appreciate Dr. Cutter's bold remarks toward me and his insensitive actions before Denise.

Dr. Cutter had to have thought his malicious actions against me would escape the watchful eye and care of the medical and dental review boards and the investigator unit. I slowly came to realize that Dr. Cutter needed to be stopped in his cosmetic tracks and the medical and dental boards needed to be warned of his insensitive actions against me.

In the nineties, I experienced an AC shoulder separation when my car did a complete rollover after losing its right rear tire. I was driving back home south of Union from my parents' place in Clover Valley, heading back to work on the highway approximately eight and a half miles outside of Granted Orchards, listening to a good Christian music station (105.3) on the radio.

As I was driving back for work during a sunny day, I heard a thud and a strange grinding noise coming from my car. I slowed down my little compact Mitsubishi automobile just a little, while turning the volume lower on my radio to listen for any noise that I initially had heard coming from my car.

As I drove along intently listening to the sound coming from my vehicle, I suddenly heard a loud braking sound as I pressed down on the brake pedal. When I braked, my car veered to the right and drove onto the gravel shoulder of the road with rapid speed. Everything became fast motion for me as I continued to apply my brake as my Mitsubishi automobile headed directly toward the embankment.

I found myself saying, "Oh, dear Jesus" as I tightly held the steering wheel. My car caught a mound of dirt at the beginning of the embankment, which caused my car to do a complete rollover and end up facing northeast. I remember that I saw stars as the dust flew high into the air around my car doing a complete rollover.

I remember that I wasn't wearing my seat belt at the time. As I remained sitting in my driver's seat, some people stopped to check if I was all right. I remember telling them that I thought I was all right, and I asked if they could call a tow truck when they got to Granted Orchards, which was the next town. They let me know that they would call for a tow truck to assist me, and they drove on from the scene of the accident.

There were other people who stopped to see if I was going to be okay, and I believed I was going to be just fine. It didn't take me too long to come to the realization that my left shoulder blade was experiencing an unusual awkward tension and it didn't feel like its normal self.

One man stopped and let me know that he had somewhere to go, but if I was still there when he came back, he would stop for me. Later, when I wasn't seeing any tow trucks coming to my location and there weren't any police or state patrol cars stopping by, I began to become concerned about my physical situation.

With darkness coming on, I remember pressing down on the brake pedal, causing my brake lights to come on and showing my whereabouts for someone to stop and help me. It was shortly after I had pushed down on my brake pedal, still sitting in the driver's seat of my Mitsubishi automobile, when I noticed a car had stopped on the shoulder of the road just over to my right. I thought that it might be the man who offered to stop back by if I was still there. By this time, I was grateful for anyone who might be of assistance to me.

Sure enough, the man who had let me know that he would stop if I was still there did a good Samaritan deed by helping me with my difficult postaccident shoulder condition. By now, I could feel that the dull knot feeling in my collarbone area was not getting any better, and the kind man offered to give me a ride to the hospital in Foggy Meadows, which was forty miles away. I accepted Ken Princeton's kind offer of a ride, and Ken drove me to the Foggy Meadows Hospital, where a medical doctor checked me for any sustained injuries.

The doctor thought it might be an AC shoulder problem, but he requested that I have two X-rays taken of my shoulder area anyway. The X-rays pretty much confirmed the doctor's suspicions, and he had me lie down while he pushed my clavicle down flush with my collarbone. I could feel the clavicle bone go back into place, and it felt perfectly fine. The medical doctor informed me that my physical condition would require having it stitched together to correct the problem.

As I was lying on the cushioned table, I thought that I was ready to go. When I got up to leave the room, I felt the clavicle bone pull away from my shoulder blade. I was given a ride to a motel, where I stayed the night taking the medications that the doctor had prescribed for my postaccident physical pain. I was grateful for the pain pills because I would have been in some real physical pain had I not had any medication during the night.

The next day, I was able to make a phone call to a car rental agency, and a representative provided a ride for me to the agency. After signing the rental agreement, I drove back to the area where I had my accident the day before. I got out of the rental car and could see the skid marks in the gravel and where my car had made contact with the side of the small hillside. I began looking for my right rear tire, which had come off my vehicle and had to be in the area somewhere. I spent some time searching for the missing tire, but I was never able to find it.

I got back into the rental car and drove to Granted Orchards, where I learned my car had been towed to. I discovered from the tow truck operator that the spindle in the center of the right rear tire had broken off. The tow truck operator was willing at my request to take out my tape player and AM-FM radio, power booster, and the speakers, all of which were still in good condition. I thanked the tow truck operator mechanic and paid him for his towing and labor services.

I once again headed for Union after driving back out to the highway. I had put a lot of miles on my Mitsubishi automobile, and I knew that I was going to have to look for another car to purchase after getting back home.

I first needed to have my shoulder problem fixed. I discovered that my surgery would take place with Dr. Harvey Crandon and Dr. Stanley Martinez at the Fairmont Medical Center in Collard.

After the two medical doctors worked on placing a metal screw to fuse my clavicle bone together with my collarbone, I was wheeled into a recovery room for the night. I remember learning that my patient roommate, who was making some painful noises on the other side of the blue partition, had had his foot crushed in eight places. I was given half of a sandwich and some juice to drink by the nurse.

As I lay in bed watching television, I kept hearing the steady aching sounds coming from my roommate. I knew I wasn't going to get any sleep hearing the continuous, disturbing sounds coming from my poor roommate. So I asked the nurse if I could be moved into a different room, where I could have some peace and quiet. The nurse had sympathy for my plight and kindly moved me into a room where I could be alone.

I found that I liked having a room by myself apart from all the moaning noise coming from my roommate. This time the nurse brought me a whole sandwich, a couple of cookies, and some more juice. I was able to relax in peace while I enjoyed my early morning meal while watching television. I discovered that I was feeling so good after having surgery that I inquired of the nurse if someone could give me a ride home. If I was going to be recovering from surgery, I might as well do it at home rather than in the hospital. The nurse informed me that there wasn't anyone available who could give me a ride. When the nurse left the room, I began thinking about walking home. It would only be a three- to four-mile walk.

As I thought on the prospects of walking home, feeling comfortable from the delicious food I had that early morning, I eventually fell asleep around four thirty in the morning.

At 7:25 a.m., I got up to use the restroom, and I began to break out into a sweat and feel faint. After using the facilities, I crawled back into bed and took a couple of the pain pills that were left for me. I came to the realization that it was a good thing that I hadn't taken off for home in the morning hours on an extremely cold winter day. The morphine that was still in my system after my clavicle surgery had shielded me from feeling the shock of really hurting in a serious way. I appreciated my decision not to leave the hospital that chilly early morning, but to wait for my ride at noon, which my good friend Leroy O'Hara would provide for me.

I appreciated having my friend Leroy sacrifice his time to come to the hospital and give me a ride home after my surgery. I had to wear a sling on my arm to protect my collarbone from pain, keep the screw safely in place, and gradually heal from my surgery, with the screw tightly fusing my AC shoulder bones together.

After healing from my surgery, I made an appointment to see Dr. Harvey Crandon to have the screw removed from my left side collarbone. When I arrived for my appointment Dr. Crandon told his receptionist, "He's been screwed, and I have to unscrew him."

I eventually returned to work after having nearly two and a half months off from work.

I made an appointment to see Dr. Cutter once more after my car accident. I was still interested in receiving a periodic cortisone injection by Dr. Cutter, who would administer it directly to my nose to facilitate the swelling or inflammation, which is in relation to neoplasty, to go down. Dr. Cutter had learned of my AC shoulder injury, and he apparently wanted to see if he could get me to become a little lighthearted regarding my cosmetic surgeries, so apparently he decided it would be a good thing to say something as a way to add a little levity to his patient's disappointment with his rhinoplasty results. When I came in to see Dr. Cutter, who was going to give me another steroid injection to help reduce the swelling in my nose, Dr. Cutter said, "Well, at least it helps to take your attention off of your nose." He then began to smile and chuckle along with his nursing assistant. I found myself lightheartedly chuckling a little along with the doctor and his female helper, who I believe was present in the consultation room to provide Dr. Cutter a witness to anything mentioned between himself and his patient.

I took mental note of Dr. Cutter's attempt to change my mental focus from being painfully obsessive thinking about my devastating rhinoplasty results. Dr. Cutter's efforts were fleetingly brief or minuscule on the scale of time; they were completely futile to me because of being totally overwhelmed and consumed by what I had experienced by the ominous character disguised as a cosmetic specialist for my nose, ears, and chin. Postsurgery I slowly came to realize that Dr. Cutter was going to have his way with his subdued patient's facial features whether I liked it or not.

The next appointment, I wanted to communicate my disappointment regarding my surgeries, and I wanted to hear what Dr. Cutter had to say about the results. When Dr. Cutter came into the room, I, who had been waiting for him, was facing sideways looking over at the lower side wall.

I was able to see Dr. Cutter take a quick look at me with my peripheral vision as he entered the room. Dr. Cutter then turned sideways, looking toward the wall, as he began to walk past me with his back facing me. I recollect that Dr. Cutter had stopped to take a look at me several feet away. As he did so, he acted like he was extremely disappointed, as if he had just missed an important hole in a game of golf.

After this, I recall sitting down at a desk across from Dr. Cutter. I said, "What happened to my nose? It looks like a turtle nose."

Dr. Cutter immediately turned around, stood up, and began looking up at the wall, with his back facing me. Dr. Cutter said, "If something could be done, we'd have to wait a year." He followed quickly with, "I hope it will come down."

The doctor finally got the courage to turn back around and to sit back down across from me once more. Dr. Cutter looked directly at me and said, "It didn't turn out as I had envisioned."

I said, "My complaint is not only that it didn't turn out as I had envisioned, but it is also with the way you went about getting my business."

I remember that Dr. Cutter just looked at me, and then he looked down as if he wanted to doodle on the table, as if he didn't even want to deal with the subject any longer. I felt that it was a good thing that I had been able to communicate with Dr. Cutter just how I felt about my cosmetic debacle. I gradually came to realize that Dr. Cutter had seriously hurt me cosmetically in the most horrifying way.

I set up an appointment to see Dr. James Evans, who had practiced in Union and then moved to Browerland. I was curious to get Dr. Evans's professional opinion regarding Dr. Cutter's postsurgery cosmetic results since he had been the plastic surgeon who had done my second rhinoplasty.

Dr. Evans took postsurgery photos of me prior to the consultation, and then said to me, "He thinks he's a plastic surgeon," referring to Dr. Cutter. Dr. Evans commented on Dr. Cutter's cosmetic work of raising the left nostril higher than normal. He said, "He didn't have to raise it that high."

When I inquired if Dr. Evans was willing to testify against Dr. Cutter, Dr. Evans declined to help me make a formal complaint against Dr. Cutter.

I could understand why Dr. Evans wouldn't want to testify against another medical doctor, especially since he continued to practice in Browerland, because most medical doctors do not like to testify against another doctor who happens to have his or her practice in the same region as the medical doctor in question.

I went to see Dr. Dwight Marshall to get his professional opinion concerning my postsurgery cosmetic results. When Dr. Marshall saw my results, he commented that he didn't know of any surgeon throughout the extended area who could be of any help to me. I called Dr. Alfred Thompson's office, a double-board plastic surgeon in Union, and he was adamant in his refusal to see me after he heard that Dr. Cutter had worked on my face.

I finally came to the understanding that I wasn't going to find any medical doctor in the surrounding area of Union and the suburbs to help me with any plastic surgery reconstructive work.

Dr. Marshall mentioned a medical surgeon in Los Angeles, who he believed could help me. Dr. Marshall gave me Dr. Raymond Rockwell's name and phone number for me to contact the doctor.

Once again, I was encouraged with new hope to continue my search for relief from my devastating cosmetic results. I looked forward to making an appointment to see Dr. Rockwell.

I had begun to explain what Dr. Cutter had done to me to a number of people who worked for cosmetic and plastic surgeons in the Union area. In the process of trying to understand why a cosmetic surgeon would move out of his medical specialty and surgically work on a multiple-surgery patient, I found out about Dr. Donald Philbert in Santa Barbara. I planned to fly down to see Dr. Philbert for a $200.00 consultation fee.

I had been informed by Kim Kincade—a nice woman who worked for a plastic surgeon in Champus—not to complain about my postsurgery results when I met with the doctor, but to see if Dr. Philbert might be able to help me. I was encouraged by what I had heard about Dr. Philbert, and I made an appointment to see him at the turn of the century.

To my disappointment, Dr. Philbert didn't think that he could help me cosmetically, although he thought he might have been able to help me provided I had come to see him before Dr. Cutter had cosmetically worked on me.

Dr. Philbert looked at my pictures, which I had brought with me in chronological order, closely examining my presurgery and postsurgery photos. He then commented to me regarding Dr. Cutter's cosmetic work, "He didn't do what you wanted." He remarked that he thought my nose looked okay for a nose job, but Dr. Philbert recognized that it wasn't what I wanted.

When I showed Dr. Philbert Dr. Cutter's business card, he responded, "He's a dentist. I don't know why a dentist would want to do it."

I left Dr. Philbert's practice and drove to Los Angeles, to see Dr. Raymond Rockwell for a separate $120.00 consultation fee.

I recall that Dr. Rockwell never said, "Hello, Kurtess. My name is Dr. Rockwell. How can I be of help to you?" Instead, Dr. Rockwell commented to me, "You're not bringing it down," making a direct reference to my elevated nose.

I was confident that Dr. Rockwell could help me by making the necessary changes to my physical characteristics based upon what I had heard about Dr. Rockwell after Dr. Cutter had disfigured and detrimentally damaged my facial features. I had learned somethings about Dr. Rockwell concerning his qualifications as a plastic surgeon, which let me know that I truly was dealing with a specialist in the nose, ears, and chin. I had met with a nice young woman who worked for Dr. Rockwell as his assistant; she shared some good information about the medical doctor with me in a private consultation room. I came to realize that Dr. Rockwell was recognized by the ABMS and is board-certified by the American Board of Plastic Surgery. He is also a specialist in the nose and ears, and as a plastic surgeon, he can also perform reconstruction for facial features. Unlike Dr. Cutter, Dr. Rockwell has the credentials and qualifications to produce good-quality cosmetic and reconstruction results for the physical enhancements that his patients come to experience and greatly appreciate.

I returned to work in Union after making the lengthy trip to see the two medical doctors in California concerning the devastating cosmetic results that Dr. Cutter had caused to my nose and ears.

I had multiple surgeries for corrective revisions on my nose, ears, and chin by Dr. Rockwell. I was not completely satisfied with my corrective revisions, and I came to realize that Dr. Rockwell was not the God of creative miracles who could make my physical characteristics completely whole and restored in their original physical image.

Dr. Rockwell had to cut under both of my breasts in order to remove cartilage to help bring my nose down from the elevated position where Dr. Cutter had placed it—against my will, expectations, and postsurgery desired results.

I had three separate corrective revisions for my physical characteristics by Dr. Rockwell, and I recognize that I am not satisfied with my current physical appearance even with all the surgeries and corrective revisions I have had.

I realize that the important rule to remember in having cosmetic or plastic surgery is to find the right qualified surgeon by first doing your homework before you ever elect to have cosmetic or plastic surgery. Learn all you can by asking a lot of questions before going in to talk with a medical surgeon.

There are some major pitfalls to avoid in searching for the right qualified surgeon for yourself that I would like the reader to know about in explicit detail. This will be discussed at a later time to help each reader know how to find the right qualified surgeon for himself or herself.

I want the reader to be informed, educated, and equipped on how to go about finding the right surgeon before he or she takes the next step of having surgery with a qualified surgeon, which will help to eliminate any future regrets like those which I have endured, survived, and had to live with.

I had so many negative thoughts coming to my mind postsurgery that I found the mental and emotional anguish was difficult for me to deal with socially, professionally, personally, and spiritually.

I told my coworker Denise that I was not pleased with my postsurgery results and was concerned about the negative thoughts I was thinking about Dr. Cutter.

Denise told me to write down my thoughts, and I came to appreciate Denise for the wise advice that my coworker had so aptly shared with me.

I ended up contacting the various medical boards with which Dr. Cutter was licensed in order to send in my complaints against him. I had slowly come to the realization that the cosmetic violations to my nose and ears were not an accident, but a cruel, callous, and cold-hearted iron will of a malicious cosmetic surgeon disguised as a medical doctor.

As the days ground mercilessly by, I became increasingly disappointed, devastated, and convinced I was victimized by a predator who cared more about gaining my cosmetic and financial business for his own professional gain and personal profits than about delivering the results that I wanted.

I went on the record and made my complaints known to each of the licensing boards Dr. Cutter was licensed with. I also sent my series of complaint letters to the state legislators in Olympia, Washington.

I would like to make my voice heard as a spokesman against medical malpractice and encourage lawmakers to change the existing laws, which benefit the predators, attorneys, judges, and legal system while the victims continue to suffer needlessly. I know beyond any shadow of a doubt that had the aforementioned experienced what I had or had any one of their family members and friends experienced it, they would also echo along with me to see that the US Congress and state legislatures throughout this great United States of America enact laws to immediately put a stop to all medical malpractice victimization in no uncertain terms in favor of the victim.

I say, "Let all medical malpractice victimization be a thing of the unfortunate, forbidden past, and positively not an active practice in these current times nor allowed in the future."

I was able to find some good definitions for medical malpractice by going to Google that could be helpful to the reader. The following definition was provided by Marlie:

> Medical malpractice is basically described as an act of extreme injury to a patient. This medical negligence shows up in different forms, such as infections cultivated

in failure to monitor the patient's vital signs, surgical errors, misdiagnosis, and failure to follow up with treatment.

I encourage the reader to contact a medical malpractice or a medical negligence lawyer or attorney if you have been a witness or a victim of either of the above.

I am an advocate to put an end to all forms of victimization through medical malpractice cases and medical negligence, whether intentional or unintentional by medical doctors and by hospitals.

I advocate that all medical doctors that are classified and categorically nonrecognized by the American Board of Plastic Surgery and the American Board of Medical Specialties remain within their respective specialization when it comes to cosmetic procedures on real patients. Doctors may consider their patients as guinea pigs, but they are real people and not paper bull's-eyes.

I recognize that medical policies must be changed now or there will be a steady stream of medical malpractice cases submitted to the medical commissions throughout Victimized, USA, and more medical boards will continuously be reviewing complaint after complaint against doctors who are suspected of committing medical malpractice crimes.

My encounter with Dr. Cutter resulted in medical malpractice assault, resulting in anguish and charges regarding my nose and ears. Such malpractice was clearly avoidable and needless if the medical boards had restricted a nonrecognized doctor with his specialty status defined and classified in dentistry, as the large letters behind his name in the yellow pages showed.

The only problem was that when I was searching for the right doctor for myself, having had previous surgeries on my nose, ears, and chin, I didn't know and I didn't understand what DDS meant—but Dr. Cutter did. Dr. Cutter should have clearly explained that his specialty was in dentistry, and not in the nose and ears. *He absolutely did not!*

I didn't know that the American Board of Cosmetic Surgery, the American Board of Oral Maxillofacial Surgery, and Board-Certified in Outpatient Surgery *was not* recognized by the ABPS, American Board of Plastic Surgery, and the ABMS, American Board of Medical Specialties, when I first encountered Dr. Cutter. When I first encountered Dr. Cutter, I didn't know what the three distinct boards above actually meant, or why these nonrecognized boards above were not accepted by the ABMS and the ABPS or how these boards had helped prepare and qualify Dr. Cutter to perform surgeries on a multisurgery patient like myself. My encounter with Dr. Cutter became a scary cosmetic nightmare for myself, physically dangerous, and painfully devastating mentally and emotionally.

I would like for the reader to be able to read for himself my complaint letters addressed to the various licensing boards and to decide whether my complaints merited having disciplinary or termination action or a criminal investigation begun against Dr. Cutter.

I would be willing to post my complaint letters, requests for a reconsideration, requests for criminal action, and legal action to be taken against Dr. Cutter, but all to no avail, on my website.

I discovered that the Medical Quality Assurance Commission, the medical board Dr. Cutter has his MD license with, and the Dental Quality Assurance Commission, which licenses Dr. Cutter's dental practice, does have an investigator unit, who determines whether a complaint merits having disciplinary or termination action taken against a medical doctor. I also learned the MQAC does not have a criminal investigator unit.

I was informed by the chief investigator, Arnold Richards, that the MQAC is the one board that authorizes reviews and investigations, and they also make the decisions.

I am convinced by what I have personally experienced and by what other medical doctors have said to me regarding Dr. Cutter's postsurgery results that I had a legitimate case, I most certainly qualified as a cosmetic and financial victim, and my case warranted having a thorough criminal investigation into Dr. Cutter's professional malpractice against me.

I recognize that when I was violated and victimized by Dr. Cutter in such a careless, ruthless, and malicious manner, I felt that I had been robbed big-time of my valuable treasures that God alone had royally given to me. It seemed totally outrageous and unexpected that a medical doctor in a position of trust had deviously ripped me off of my priceless possessions through mental manipulation and nonrecognized surgical procedures on my facial features. I was trying to be so careful about choosing the right surgeon for my special cosmetic needs before I gave my permission to the surgeon to correct my facial features with precision in detail and skilled surgical care. When I least expected it, in a secluded dark room, an unqualified medical thief, Dr. Cutter, decided to rob me while I was on the road of finding a qualified specialist in the nose, ears, and chin. I am authorizing the lawful authorities mentioned in this book to find the notorious thief named Dr. Cutter and carry out the true prevailing justice against the dishonest thief, the notable criminal described and found guilty of crimes committed against me. I leave the legal prosecution of Dr. Cutter to the above authorities since I was never able to bring a lawsuit against him myself.

Dr. Cutter referred me to see Dr. Salmon Pride for consultation because he became aware that I felt seriously hurt by Dr. Cutter's actions against me. Dr. Cutter also informed me that sometimes we need to receive counseling, which can be of help during difficult times.

When I went to see Dr. Pride, he looked tired, and he wasn't saying anything as he sat in a chair remaining silent, possibly gathering his thoughts.

Dr. Pride responded to my disappointment with my cosmetic results by saying, "There was a woman who had her nose worked on the second time, and it was worse than before. I won't say it wasn't Dr. Cutter."

Dr. Pride didn't think he could help me regarding doing something for me cosmetically, but looking back, I feel that the short time I spent with the kind doctor was a good thing in hindsight. I appreciated talking to Dr. Pride postsurgery as a referred consultant recommended by Dr. Cutter, and in retrospect, I think Dr. Pride was giving me information to use should I bring a case against Dr. Cutter or report him to the proper authorities.

I didn't have the mental wherewithal postsurgery to do much other than suffer needlessly day in and day out. It was a slow, agonizing, painful process that I was forced to endure and suffer through as I wrote down my negative thoughts toward Dr. Cutter. I eventually began to send in my complaints, which I had patiently prepared, to the licensing boards.

Although I was experiencing mental difficulties postsurgery, I continuously took the time to write down what I could remember Dr. Cutter had done to me. I was confident that the medical review board would take disciplinary action against Dr. Cutter upon receiving my complaints, but I found out later they never did.

When I discovered the Medical Quality Assurance Commission hadn't even required Dr. Cutter to respond to my complaints, I couldn't believe their inaction when I knew that Dr. Cutter had committed sinister criminal actions against me. I continued to suffer mercilessly personally, socially, and professionally as the days rolled slowly and agonizingly by.

The consequences of my personal encounter with Dr. Cutter dramatically, drastically, and negatively impacted my performance in my profession and the quality of my personal life.

My professional and personal life had been devastated by the harmful cosmetic results of the surgeries performed by Dr. Cutter and by the cold reaction I received from the general public. After my horrifying experience, I didn't feel safe to pursue corrective surgeries with Dr. Cutter.

I have appreciated my coworkers and every person who has shown me acceptance in society with my physical imperfections. I have tried to rise above the negative reactions by a lot of passengers who ride my carrier routes. Due to embarrassing cosmetic results caused by the careless handiwork of a nonrecognized cosmetic surgeon, I have been left to deal with many difficult situations on the job and in life in general.

I also experienced negative reactions from people in the Christian churches when they observed my adverse physical characteristics.

As a negative outcome of Dr. Cutter's surgical actions, I have been dealing with victimization by self-centered people in society in spite of having attempted corrective surgeries with Dr. Raymond Rockwell. I am not giving in to society's pressure, expressed through various tactics of many passengers, to give up driving my personnel carrier routes. Postsurgery, I found that the general public had difficulty looking at my new physical look, and I also found certain people looking or staring at me, and then suddenly looking away in haste when I would look in their direction. I had a carrier driver looking intently at my new appearance at the work site, and when I perceived he was staring at me, I quickly tried to move away from being stared at. I had customers, clients, and passengers on my personnel carriers showing by their uneasy actions that they were uncomfortable being on my carrier. They seemed to have difficulty looking in my direction, and so I would find different ones looking at a door to exit my carrier vehicle only to swiftly dart off my carrier in a rapid manner without saying good-bye or even a thoughtful "thank you, driver." Postsurgery, I found that many people weren't as friendly or accepting of me as presurgery attitudes, manners of courtesy, and acceptable social etiquette standards mandated. Unaware of what I would be left to deal with on my social plate, my performance on my carrier routes and in difficult social settings has been reduced by adverse gossip.

Overall, society shows a lack of concern for my feelings. Social interactions prove that I am an object of ridicule through deliberate ignorance on society's part.

I have chosen to be a man of principle over popularity. I have decided to weather the storms of social rejections and adversities and withstand the pressures of persistent objections to see the good that comes to those who persevere through the stormy winds of opposition. In fact, I actually thank God for His love and grace to endure and persevere through the storms of social opposition, resistance, and rejections by the general public. I remember my friend Sean Ridpath saying, "I'm like mold. I grow on you." Through many years of safe, friendly, and courteous driving service, I have come to adopt a philosophical attitude regarding the passengers who pull a conspicuous absence toward riding my personnel carrier: "Let them come, and let them go."

I remember my mother, Jessica, making a remark concerning company who would come for a visit to the Scone family residence: "I like the comers and goers. Not the comers and stayers."

I recognize that God always causes those who place their faith and trust in Him, the Lord Jesus Christ, to triumph through tough times, difficult situations, and every unpleasant circumstance. Glory to God for his victorious intervention in the face of tough situations that Christians face in this life.

I would like for the reader to take a look at the letter Dr. Cutter sent me recommending a consultation with Dr. Pride and to seek out some counseling help:

June 5th, 1997

Mr. Kurtess Scone
00000 0000 000., So.
City, WA. 00000

Dear Kurtess:

This letter is a follow-up to your recent post-operative visit in my office Wednesday 6/4/97. As you know, you had a 5:00 appointment. We had you stay in the library until Cindy seated you at approximately 5:30, at which time she took images. I spent from approximately 5:45 to 6:45 with you in consultation in the imaging room. It should also be noted I examined you clinically in one of the exam rooms with particular attention paid to the nasal exam.

Examination that day and review of the images show the following findings:

1. The chin is healing well with good position, though the patient is somewhat concerned about some asymmetry. However, the full beard makes it difficult to judge the symmetry at this time.
2. There is still a small patch of resolving alopecia on the chin and some minor skin irregularity over the corrected crease in the chin. The patient was told that there probably will be further resorption of the area, and most likely the alopecia will continue to resolve itself.
3. Good position of the ears with some very minor asymmetry. Overall, improvement was noted with regards to their position.
4. Intranasal examination showed a patient airway on both sides. The patient reports somewhat restricted airflow on the left side. Some scar tissue was noted in the left anterior nose that may be contributing to some of the airflow issues. The nasal mucosa was noted to be slightly erythematous.
5. External nasal examination showed the nose to be healing well with good overall symmetry. There still is some fullness in the nasal tip which is to be expected at this relatively early post-operative point.

Kurtess, I spent approximately 1 hour with you and Denise in the imaging room as we reviewed and discussed your progress. You had some concerns that the tip had been lifted up somewhat, however I pointed out that your tip was still swollen. This is very normal post-operatively, particularly for someone who has had 2 previous rhinoplasties to the one that I did. A large part of your concern seems to resolve around the augmentation of the dorsum. You told me that I only discussed this with you on the day of surgery. I pointed out to you in my progress notes which *were dictated at our initial consultation in February 1997, that I clearly delineated that your dorsum was over-reduced and that part of my treatment plan was to augment the dorsum. If somehow I failed to communicate that to you clearly at that time, I sincerely apologize. However, I also showed you the changes on the computer imaging which I had done for you at your initial consult. The images clearly indicated that I had treatment planned for you to have the dorsum built-up. Again, I apologize if there was any misunderstanding.*

Over the last two months you have been concerned about your appearance. I know that you have seen at least two of my colleagues for consultation with regard to your early surgical results. You expressed your concerns to them and both of them have indicated that you are doing well and have no significant problems. You are certainly free to see anyone you wish with regard to your surgical outcomes, however I would have appreciated being informed about your specific concerns. I feel I could have been of more assistance with regard to your issues. After our discussion on Wednesday, I do not believe that you are satisfied with your surgical outcome to date. I would encourage you to seek further consultation. One individual that I would recommend that you see is Dr. Salmon Pride. He has a national reputation for lecturing on nasal surgery and is very well respected in this community. In order to facilitate this, I have enclosed a copy of your pre and post-operative photographs in case you will need them. I would also encourage you to have Dr. Pride call me so that I can discuss your case with him (with your permission, of course).

With regard to giving your money back, I believe that was an inappropriate request. You are progressing well in your post-surgical course. Two other surgeons have stated that to be true and I have stated that to be true. I will be glad to remain your doctor and do everything I can to help with the healing process.

Finally, Kurtess, I am concerned about your over-scrutiny of yourself. It is not normal to have a one hour post-operative visit that you were "totally devastated" over the last few months because of your surgery. Three highly qualified surgeons have looked at you and all have said you are healing well. I would be remiss as a physician not to be deeply concerned about this situation, and therefore I am recommending that you seek some counseling help in order to deal with some of your concerns. Kurtess, please don't take this recommendation in a negative way. All of us need someone to talk to at some point in our lives. I am very concerned about you and I believe that counseling would be of benefit for you.

I hope this letter helps clarify some of the issues. I will continue to be your doctor. Kurtess, I like you as an individual and I hope that we can work together in the future. I did tell you that I would like to see you in 1 month for further follow-up care and evaluation and you agreed to make that appointment. Again, thank you for your attention to this letter. I look forward to seeing you in early July.

Sincerely,

Thadeaus D. Cutter, MD

TDC:dc

―――――

At the turn of the century, I sent in a complaint against Dr. Cutter; it turned out to be only the first in a series of complaints. I was so devastated by Dr. Cutter's mental and cosmetic violations against me that I sent in a volume of paperwork to the medical boards instead of one or two pages because I felt I needed to prove my case against Dr. Cutter with substantial, hard-hitting evidence that I clearly was victimized, although I found that I wasn't able to pinpoint the exact moment of my victimization until years later.

With all the convincing evidence I could supply, I was doing my level best to persuade the medical and dental review teams to take disciplinary or termination action against Dr. Cutter.

I threw Dr. Cutter a negative curveball when I sent in my critical thoughts to the medical and dental review boards as to the predatory treatment that I had experienced at the hands of Dr. Cutter. I decided to use my sharp cutting ax, expressed in my negative word pictures utilizing numerous illustrations as to the way I saw Dr. Cutter.

I also tried to warn the medical and dental boards that they had a dangerous medical doctor on their boards who would end up hurting other unsuspecting patients—and he has—if his predatory cosmetic practice was not stopped.

I sent in a series of complaint letters to the different licensing boards Dr. Cutter was licensed with, and to Shay Schual-Berke, a legislator in the House of Representatives in Olympia, Washington, against Dr. Cutter in November.

I was making the trip over to see my parents in the early fall one year when a young deer suddenly darted out from the side of the road and ran into the left side of my car. After I was able to get my automobile stopped from traveling at a good rate of speed, I managed to turn my car around in the dark of the early morning hours. I turned on my bright headlights, and I could clearly see the deer lying down on the shoulder of the road.

I thought for sure that I had killed the deer when I saw it lying there without movement. I got out of my vehicle to take a closer look, and I noticed that the deer's side was going up and down with every breath he managed to take. I observed white spots all over its body, and I realized the deer was a fawn that had taken a hard hit when it ran directly into my car.

I placed my hand on the young deer's side, and I prayed for the Lord to heal it and raise it up. As I kept praying for the fawn, it eventually raised its head, and I could see blood on the mouth and nose of the animal. I petted the deer as I again prayed for the creature to be healed and to enjoy the life that God had created it for.

I continued to pray for the young deer to be healed, and after a while, it finally was able to stand up with my assistance. The fawn was still stunned from the trauma of hitting its muzzle above the left front wheel wall of my vehicle.

I was pleased to see the deer making gradual progress in response to my prayers for the four-legged animal; the Lord God was helping the fawn to make a full recovery from its stunning collision with the fast-moving car.

For years, I had made the lengthy drive over to spend time with my parents in Clover Valley, by taking the highway north to travel east on I-90 through the Snoqualmie Pass and beyond. After I drove across the

Sacajawea River bridge, I would continue heading east on the highway until I reached another little town. I have found that there are a lot of small towns in the state of Washington. After driving through Donny Brook Lair on my long highway travels, I came to the turning point that would take me homeward to Clover Valley; that was the location where the fawn had unfortunately run into my car.

God had answered my prayers for the young deer, and it tried to make it across a ditch. The deer fell on the knoll on the other side of the ditch, and it lay there momentarily. As I contemplated helping the fawn continue on its journey, the deer managed to regain some extra strength and make it through a barbed wire fence to the other side.

As the deer stood in the tall yellow weeds in the field, it looked back at me as if to take one last look at a good Samaritan who had taken time to help a wounded friend in the battle of life. Once again, God gets the glory for answering prayer and coming through to facilitate the life of one of His creatures.

I got back on the road again and made it to the Scone family home. Once inside my parents' home, I contacted the Price Police Department to see if a fish and game ranger could go out to the location that I described where I last saw the deer and check on its well-being. I later found out that a ranger had gone out to check on the young deer, and it was never observed in the surrounding area, which was a good sign that it had fully recovered.

Social suffering for years as a consequence of misdirected cosmetic surgeries should not be necessary because of medical doctors who show a lapse in good judgment when performing cosmetic procedures on real people. Especially if the patient has had previous surgeries on the face area, as I had on my nose, ears, and chin, precision quality cosmetic procedures with subtle minimal changes to a patient's physical appearance is in the patient's best interest and should be the positive goal and result of a doctor's work.

No patient in his or her right mind wants to ignorantly encounter a buzz saw, a butcher, or a nonrecognized cosmetic surgeon who is not specialized in the nose and ears, especially when he or she has had previous surgeries on the nose, ears, and chin.

I am willing to go on the record by saying, "From a patient's perspective, I recognize that any nonrecognized cosmetic surgeon willing to do some additional cutting on a multiple-surgery patient is a full-fledged criminal, butcher, and money-greedy predator."

The medical commissions throughout Victimized, USA, must stop this nonsensical madness and stop turning a blind eye or looking away from the growing horror of medical malpractice. Real people are being hurt by medical doctors and by hospital negligence. Real people are being victimized by self-interested medical doctors, and many patients die each year as a painful reminder of this serious subject.

The legislators, medical commissions, medical doctors, and attorneys must recognize that there are predators disguised as medical doctors who want you to accept the erroneous notion that all patients who negatively complain about being victimized by a doctor are simply mental hypochondriacs trying to smear a good doctor's reputation. After all, it's the patient's fault he or she got hurt in the first place.

"A fan assaulted violently by a baseball bat-wielding thug is at fault simply because he or she attended a baseball game? I don't think so! This same principle applies to a patient encountering a medical doctor in a position of trust, and being maliciously victimized as a consequence of encountering the wrong medical doctor and cosmetic surgeon motivated by greed, power, and self interests," as shared with me by my friend Bud, aka, Brutus Knuckles.

I would like for the reader to draw his or her own conclusions regarding medical malpractice taking place in the United States of America and reach a verdict, as I have, that medical malpractice is a blight on society that must be stopped immediately.

As a positive consequence of my painful encounter with the wrong cosmetic surgeon for myself, I have come up with a plan to help change and put a stop to this horrifying threat to so many innocent lives.

I found that it was a long, slow, and painful process for me to solve the criminal actions taken by Dr. Cutter against me. I realize that it's one thing to be viewed by other people as an oddity or as a freak of nature and thus be ostracized, discriminated against, and left out of feeling warmly accepted for who I am as a human being. It's quite another thing to be coldly rejected because of misdirected cosmetic procedures that leave an unsuspecting patient physically disfigured and cosmetically damaged due to the self-interests of an uncaring cosmetic surgeon.

I realize that I have been a social enigma to many people throughout the years. Dr. Cutter discovered that I was not hypersuggestible nor

THE ULTIMATE VIOLATION

hypnotically programmable postsurgery regarding the devastating cosmetic changes to my nose, ears, and chin.

I was unwillingly and willfully cosmetically violated by a nonspecialized cosmetic surgeon. I came to the realization that I was run over roughshod by a cosmetic predator utilizing devious, sinister, and criminal tactics.

How could I support this fact with solid evidence? I sent in my complaints to the different medical boards complaining about Dr. Cutter's dishonest and dishonorable approach taken with me. The various medical and dental boards Dr. Cutter is licensed with corresponded with me by repeatedly informing me they were not going to take any disciplinary action against Dr. Cutter. They also did not open a criminal investigation against Dr. Cutter, as I had requested. I discovered this after nearly seven years of making my requests and appeals for some type of action to be taken against Dr. Cutter, all to no avail. I received a letter informing me for the last time that the Medical Quality Assurance Commission (MQAC) was not going to reopen my request for a reconsideration.

I learned that the MQAC had already decided not to take any action as to my request after one or two years from the date of my first complaint. The medical board had not informed me of this ruling up front, and I thought I still had a chance of having my request honored and granted for a reconsideration against Dr. Cutter up to the last day for appeals.

TRAPPED BY A PSYCHO DOCTOR

The cosmetic changes that negatively impacted my facial features were horrifying and painfully devastating to my self-image and self-esteem. The negative reactions to my new appearance by the general public were very judgmental and cold.

I came to believe that the cosmetic changes to my facial characteristics were not an accident. When I sent in a series of complaint letters to the different boards that the cosmetic surgeon was licensed with, they never required the medical doctor to respond to my complaints. I couldn't understand why the boards didn't take disciplinary action against the surgeon who messed up my facial features.

The cosmetic changes were completely opposite of what I wanted, needed, and expected specifically for my nose and ears. The cosmetic surgeon copped out by responding to my complaints with, "He has psychological issues." In my mind, this brusque analysis by the surgeon regarding my cosmetic violations didn't come close to the horrible mental and emotional anguish I was facing on a daily basis.

The devastating deviations to my cosmetic blueprint were too glaringly pronounced for them to be mere trivial slips of the doctor's cosmetic knife. I, slowly came to the realization that I had been victimized without mercy by a cosmetic butcher. As the days and weeks ground mercilessly by, I continuously reflected on my cosmetic experience at the hands of the nonrecognized cosmetic surgeon. I pondered the different remarks and comments communicated to me and to others by the cosmetic surgeon.

Postsurgery, Dr. Thadeaus Damon Cutter stated to me, "See it as a sculpture. I tore it down, beat it up, and built it back up."

Dr. Cutter never mentioned anything concerning this cosmetic plan of action presurgery to me. If that was the medical doctor's cosmetic agenda, why hadn't he clearly communicated this up front with me?

The cosmetic surgeon, MD, DDS, thought that I might have psychological issues because my coworker Denise, in whom I often confided, shared with Dr. Cutter that I had difficulty going out into public settings postsurgery.

Was this response by the cosmetic surgeon to the boards an accurate evaluation of my mental perception of my facial features, or something more sinister in nature by Dr. Cutter as a smoke screen to cover his predatory actions against me? Did the cosmetic damages occur to my nose and ears because of my persistent obsession with my physical appearance, or were they caused by the unskilled actions of a cosmetic predator?

The lines had become blurred in my mind by what I had experienced at the hands of the cosmetic surgeon presurgery. I suffered needlessly postsurgery because one cosmetic surgeon forged strongly ahead, plundering my cosmetic and financial business. I was left confused, numb, and perplexed as to what had actually happened to me mentally and cosmetically because of the nonrecognized cosmetic surgeon.

My postsurgery suffering would continue for years despite three corrective revision surgeries for my nose and ears by a renowned, board-certified plastic surgeon. I know now for a 100 percent fact that Dr. Cutter absolutely did not rightly interpret my cosmetic wants and needs, and by the actions and words communicated to me postsurgery, Dr. Cutter didn't think that I would have a strong, accurate recollection of details.

I came to the realization that I had been violated by a cosmetic predator, violator, and butcher. *How would I ever prove it to the licensing boards?* I tried to warn the boards by which Dr. Cutter was licensed that if I had been seriously hurt by the nonrecognized cosmetic surgeon, then Dr. Cutter would hurt other unsuspecting consumers for professional gain and personal profit.

I found out sometime later that the boards never required Dr. Cutter to respond to my complaints. What an outrage and an insult to me!

I came to the realization that I was powerless to stop the cosmetic surgeon from making painfully scary changes to my facial features. I recognized that the board-certified plastic surgeon Dr. Raymond Rockwell, while doing his very best to make positive cosmetic revisions for me, was not able to perform creative miracles concerning my nose and ears. Painful cosmetic damages and violations had already been made by the nonrecognized cosmetic surgeon that the board-certified plastic surgeon couldn't eliminate nor undo.

I had spoken to a nice woman who works for a recognized plastic surgeon in Union. The woman informed me that Dr. Cutter tells people that he is triple-board certified. A plastic surgeon who practices in Browerland told me that Dr. Cutter thinks he is a plastic surgeon. I realize that I may think of myself as a rocket scientist or as a presidential candidate, but I would never take steps of action to place myself into a position of being a rocket scientist for NASA nor as the next president of the United States. If I were to place myself in either position, I could cause a lot of damage in various ways that could hurt a lot of innocent people.

I came to the inevitable conclusion that Dr. Cutter knew the system that the boards work with, and so he did everything possible to avoid detection by abusing an unsuspecting consumer. My personal and social life was devastated and literally destroyed by a sociopathic cosmetic surgeon.

Dr. Cutter was communicating things to me postsurgery that he absolutely did not communicate to me presurgery. This was clearly a case of abnormal psychology that I endured without mentally detecting it. Dr. Cutter knew precisely what he was going to do in each step of the cosmetic approach that he utilized on me without my consent. I didn't have a clue what the cosmetic surgeon might have in store for me presurgery.

I was naïve in my attempt to understand exactly what the cosmetic surgeon was not communicating, but I positively didn't deserve to be treated in such a ruthless and abusive manner by the medical doctor—especially when the medical doctor has taken a sacred oath to not do anything that would compromise the trust of every citizen under his care.

I recognize that had any board member experienced what I underwent at the hands of Dr. Cutter, the board member would positively make a judgment ruling that truly this was a cosmetic and financial crime.

I now know conclusively that I was trapped by a psycho doctor in his presurgery, dimly lit room.

Dr. Cutter wanted me to be a blank slate, a mental basket case, and he especially wanted for me to act the part of a psychological specimen of radical, nonrecognized cosmetic changes.

Dr. Cutter knew exactly when to catch me mentally off guard to psychologically deceive and dupe me into believing that my extreme cosmetic changes were merely my own erroneous psychological issues.

The steady stream of social and professional rejections was abusive and personally destructive to my wholeness as a person.

I worked on isolating myself from group and social settings. I had a sad case of inferiority complex and a worse case of feeling totally inadequate in terms of looking and feeling normal. I had so much stress because of the post-traumatic cosmetic violations to my cosmetic wants and needs. It may have been like pulling teeth without administering anesthesia by the nonrecognized cosmetic surgeon, but I know for a 100 percent fact that many cosmetic clients would have killed themselves had they been subjects of painful, devastating cosmetic violations to their God-given facial features. Without God's saving grace to sustain a cosmetic victim, many may resort to the unthinkable and unredeemable act of self-murder.

Cosmetic surgeons who commit criminal acts of cosmetic violations may like to put a lot of distance between themselves and their cosmetic crimes and deeds, but no crime is 100 percent perfect. The medical community is filled with psychotic doctors who are extremely intelligent, but they are not necessarily in touch with the needs and feelings of their cosmetic consumers. Many of these medical doctors live in their own ivory tower of narcissistic fantasies of grandiose power, control, and invincibility. These medical doctors think that they will get away with their cosmetic crimes. The review boards may repeatedly turn a deaf ear to the consumers' pleas for a criminal investigation if they can't come up with the winning combination as to what may have exactly happened to them pre- and during surgery.

My cosmetic surgeon waited until the actual day of surgery to psychologically take over and cosmetically do the unthinkable and unimaginable on my nose and ears. My cosmetic concerns meant absolutely nothing to Dr. Cutter presurgery, and he didn't even have a good answer postsurgery for the cosmetic deviations he had made to my facial features.

The cosmetic surgeon had conquered me psychologically presurgery, and he was on a power trip postsurgery until his subdued victim began to question what had happened to him. I had no partial or full understanding in Dr. Cutter's presurgery, dimly lit room. I was clearly communicating to the cosmetic surgeon in the conscious realm, and Dr. Cutter wanted to make cosmetic changes after he had totally neutralized and impaired his subdued victim's mental faculties in the unconscious dimension. The nonrecognized plastic surgeon was making a call for changes on the day of surgery as a quarterback of a professional football team would call for a change of play at the line of scrimmage.

Presurgery, Dr. Cutter said, "I'm going to raise and reposition your nose." It would take me a long, painful process to come to the realization years after my surgeries just how Dr. Cutter's call came for the changes he was going to make after he had utilized hypnotic paralysis to neutralize my brain, so with me as his subdued patient, he could have total control of my cosmetic outcome.

Postsurgery, while I was waking up from surgery still on the table, Dr. Cutter said, "You're going to like it." I was not hypersuggestible to Dr. Cutter's hypnotic suggestion postsurgery as the doctor was expecting.

I want the good people of Victimized, USA, to know that it was not my doing to alter my appearance completely opposite of my wants and needs cosmetically.

My wife, Lorena, wondered why I did not leave my nose just the way it looked in my presurgery photo. After all, I was only interested in having minor subtle changes done to my nose to improve its overall appearance, instead of experiencing major drastic changes caused as a dire consequence of Dr. Cutter's surgical actions. I explained to my spouse that I would have left my nose just the way it looked presurgery, had Dr. Cutter not forged ahead causing drastic, scary violations to my nose and ears, and had I known that Dr. Cutter was not the specialist in the nose and ears I was searching for presurgery. I was still seeking specific detailed information from Dr. Cutter to satisfy my questions that we were on the same page cosmetically and he could fulfill the specific qualifications with precision skill in order to exercise the surgical rights to meet the conditions of my desired results notes, which the doctor had a copy of. Unfortunately Dr. Cutter decided to totally skip the dialogue regarding my notes and whether he could or couldn't do what I was wanting and needing. After Dr. Cutter had subdued me mentally through hypnosis, the cosmetic surgeon took over and forced changes on my nose and ears that were totally against my will and cosmetic interests. Dr. Cutter completely misinterpreted my cosmetic blueprint for my nose and ears.

Dr. Donald Philbert's evaluation of Dr. Cutter's cosmetic work on me stated, "The miscommunication with the oral surgeon was sad."

Dr. Raymond Rockwell said to me, "I see a lot of poor results. A lot of poor results."

I have suffered immeasurably postsurgery to an extent that is inconceivable to the general public. Average citizens judge my appearance while not having any understanding that when they look at me, they are witnesses of criminal cosmetic changes that were totally out of my control.

Dr. Raymond Rockwell performed heroic cosmetic revisions on my nose and ears, but he could only do so much to reverse the disfigurement caused by the nonrecognized cosmetic surgeon.

I requested a criminal investigation by the review boards against Dr. Cutter, but they refused to take action against him. I know that Dr. Cutter should have served prison time for the false representation of his credentials and for the cosmetic violations to my nose and ears. Dr. Cutter knew full well before he started to make cosmetic changes on me that he was not a board-certified plastic surgeon. I didn't know this when I came in to see Dr. Cutter during our first, second, or even third consultation.

The reader may think that I was naïve for not doing my homework before seeing cosmetic and plastic surgeons in hopes of finding the right surgeon for myself. Dr. Cutter did not allow me to continue my search. He took charge of my innocent naïveté and literally trapped me in his dimly lit, presurgery, hypnotic room. It took me years to completely figure out what the medical review boards were looking for to bring disciplinary action or criminal charges against Dr. Cutter. I had been trapped and victimized by a ruthless and uncaring cosmetic surgeon.

I believe that medical predators are able to recognize their potential victims and seem to know when and how to strike. In their field they have learned how to hide themselves beyond the reach of the law and away from the criminal justice system.

"Predators typically cloak themselves with treachery in order to avoid being detected and arrested. People who call in complaints are made to look like a drooling bamboozled hypochondriac," as my friend Bud told me.

I was an innocent victim of a psychopathic mastermind disguised as a medical doctor, who wanted to advance his cosmetic credentials and medical career into an accelerated position far beyond his cosmetic training.

Dr. Cutter thought that it was necessary to skip the detailed dialogue with me and quickly place me into a mental state where I would have no recourse of changing my mind concerning the cosmetic changes Dr. Cutter was about to make on me.

I know unequivocally that Dr. Cutter wasn't going to allow me to say no to the totally inappropriate and unnecessary cosmetic changes he was going to have forced onto my facial features.

I want the reader to know that there is a big difference between a board-certified plastic surgeon and a nonrecognized, board-certified cosmetic surgeon. There is an even bigger difference if the plastic surgeon is double-board certified and has training in the specific facial feature that you desire cosmetic improvement for. Cosmetic surgeons may be able to perform the same cosmetic procedure that the board-certified plastic surgeon can do, but if the reader is a multiple-surgery cosmetic patient, you may experience dire results caused by a medical surgeon's negligence that can be destructive to your physical appearance.

I was searching for the right plastic or cosmetic surgeon who could cosmetically do exactly what I needed and wanted for my nose and ears. Dr. Cutter wasn't going to permit me to continue my search. Instead, he decided to utilize mental trickery and thuggery against me to advance his professional statistics in regard to his professional gain and personal profits. Dr. Cutter's professional tactics negatively changed my physical characteristics in the nineties.

The nature of my job demanded daily contact with multitudes of paying public customers. The true impact of those cosmetic violations to my nose and ears led to years of professional and social rejections by my fellow carrier drivers and customers. The hurtful cosmetic deviations led to years of negative impact upon my abilities to function in a professional, courteous manner.

I recognize that there are professionals in different fields of practice who have a slipshod attitude where they do not service the customer regarding the specifications as to exactly what the consumer wants and needs and what the consumer expects to be paying for. This situation applies across the board to the medical field as well.

My father, Benjamin, was a wonderful barber. He was an old-school barber who hadn't kept up with all the new barber schooling techniques that can provide tailor-made specification haircuts. His customers appreciated his barbering expertise with finesse, which resulted in many satisfied returning customers. He never needed every new barbering technique to deal with the demands and expectations of our modern society. Benjamin had naturally gifted barbering talent and honed razor-cutting skills that had been perfected over the years by a lot of practice.

I know that my father had many customers because he had excellent barbering skills and used precision care for each of his consumers. I recognize, on the other hand, that there are some barbers who, regardless of what the customer's instructions may be concerning his or her specific haircut needs, due to a lack of proper barber training skills, these barbers may get the unsuspecting consumer's haircut needs wrong in many cases.

We all know that a person's hair will eventually grow back if his or her haircut turns out to be a disaster, but a person's facial feature debacle cannot expect the same good fortune. Be cautious of barbers, medical doctors, and all professionals. Never assume that all professionals will always get it right according to your specifications and that the results will always be to your liking.

To use an old Roman phrase, "Let the buyer beware."

I recognize that I ran into a medical doctor who was on a power trip where it's what the doctor orders that matters, not what the patient orders and expects. Dr. Cutter and all other delusional-thinking doctors who are on a power trip are willing to run a slipshod cosmetic and financial business if need be to get the patient's business at all costs. Even if the unsuspecting consumer gets hurt in the process, these power trippers are going to have things done their way. The patient is forced to accept whatever the doctor has ordered. No medical doctor would intentionally wait until the actual day of surgery to catch an unsuspecting cosmetic consumer mentally off guard unless he fully doesn't care about the patient's cosmetic interests and expectations—and he positively for a 100 percent fact does not care about the patient as an individual.

I know that what I experienced at the hands of Dr. Cutter was nothing short of a cosmetic and financial heist, with evidence of a sinister crime.

Based upon firsthand factual experience, I know that Dr. Cutter is not specialized in the nose and ears. Dr. Cutter's specialized training is in dentistry—he is a DDS—and I know explicitly that a dentist without being a certified American Board Plastic Surgeon absolutely should not be surgically performing cosmetic procedures on me, who he fully knows is a multiple-surgery patient for the nose, ears, and chin. I have discovered that a Certified American Board Plastic Surgery medical doctor has undergone specialized training in reconstructive surgery for patients' faces. Dr. Cutter was certainly aware of the fact that he had not undergone such specialized training.

I know for an absolute fact due to my personal experiences that delusional-thinking medical doctors are slackers who will not mentally wake up until they have been confronted negatively regarding their irresponsibility. I know that every delusional-thinking medical doctor is a slacker when it comes to the specialized medical training that the Certified American Board of Plastic Surgery medical doctors have to complete and the specialized training that they are required to undergo.

I know for an absolute fact that I was clearly victimized by Dr. Cutter's irresponsible actions regarding my specific cosmetic needs. I recognize that until victims just like myself are willing to become negative by complaining to the medical boards and standing firm regarding our legitimate complaints, the victimization will continue in Victimized, USA. Now is the time to let all victims, friends of victims, and potential victims forever be willing to make our voices heard by taking a firm stand against victimization of our fellow men and women; we must answer a swift call to action to put an end to all forms of victimization in Victimized, USA, and Victimized, World.

I recognize now that Dr. Cutter utilized mental trickery and thuggery to plunder my cosmetic and financial business. In order to achieve this, he needed to ultimately deceive me and, once again, the medical boards in his professional career. I discovered postsurgery that I was not the only one hurt by Dr. Cutter.

Medical doctors who are not recognized by the American Board Certification of Plastic Surgery know that they are on a power-trip express train with a one-way ticket to cosmetic derailment with unsuspecting consumers' cosmetic expectations, but they will not stop their express train because there is big money to be made along the way. The only successful way to stop these power trippers is for the medical boards to stop their extracurricular cosmetic surgeries on all multiple-surgery cosmetic consumers. Without the medical boards' restrictions placed upon these power-hungry medical doctors, the patient will continue to pay the ultimate price cosmetically and financially. These power trippers must be stopped at all costs.

I am convinced that Dr. Cutter quickly moved me to surgery in an manipulative manner not only as a professional status maker for himself, but as a way to signify that he had ultimately conquered, deceived, and achieved the pinnacle of true cosmetic success as a cosmetic slacker who had cut corners regarding the extra training that board-certified plastic surgeons undergo.

My former brother-in-law, Randell Wikum, is now serving time in Lurch State Penitentiary for killing his wife. He is now under the watchful eye of Warden Crunch. Whenever I tried to get one over on Randell, he would always do his level best to top whatever I did to him. In the same way, I know now that Dr. Cutter ignored all of my cosmetic wants, needs, and expectations, believing he could manipulate me into accepting his cosmetic agenda postsurgery and I would not be the wiser for it. The effects from this mental manipulation would have long-lasting consequences for me.

Any medical doctor cruel enough to utilize this painful, mentally stunning tactic that Dr. Cutter used on me is a true predator from my perspective. The mental and emotional anguish that I suffered miserably was way beyond the scope of Dr. Cutter's calculated, insensitive, and cruel comments postsurgery. If Dr. Cutter had come across as a sensitive and caring cosmetic surgeon pre- and post-surgery, he might have been able to pull off his cosmetic and financial heist against me. On the contrary, based on the facts and solid evidence, Dr. Cutter's approach that he took toward me was cruel, criminal, and immoral. In the right hands, plastic and cosmetic surgery can be an art of facial and physical enhancement and beauty. In the wrong surgical hands, cosmetic surgery can be scary, painfully devastating, and mentally and emotionally abusive.

I recall going to have my hair cut one afternoon at Supercuts in Fedora Fair. The barber giving me a haircut asked me what kind of work I did. I told the barber that I was a carrier operator.

I reflected back on why the barber would ask me such a personal question when I hadn't had a haircut by this particular man before. I concluded the reason had to be motivated by my physical appearance, primarily my nose and ears, which have an unusual look. There is always a possibility that the barber is naturally nosy and uses the opportunity to get to know his clients by asking personal questions concerning their line of employment. My mind-set at the time made me think the barber's direct approach with me was to gain an understanding as to why my physical characteristics had such a different look about them, which to the physical eye was out of the ordinary.

I recognize that I didn't have any choice in the family planning when my parents decided to have children. Dr. Cutter didn't give me a choice in the matter regarding my cosmetic destination. Once he took charge of my cosmetic destination on the day of surgery back in the nineties, I was cut out of my cosmetic blueprint by Dr. Cutter. I have suffered and continues to suffer. I want to reach a point in life where the suffering of professional and social rejections and humiliating and embarrassing situations will forever end. This may be an unrealistic impossibility in an ever-increasingly cold and indifferent world. I can continue to look to my Creator, the Good Shepherd, to give me faith and hope for creative miracles for my nose and ears. I know that nothing is impossible with my wonderful God.

Before readers ever begin their search for the right cosmetic or plastic surgeon for themselves, they will want to read *The Ultimate Violation*. I am living testimony against a malicious cosmetic predator who had disguised himself as a caring medical surgeon. Dr. Cutter has an Outpatient Board Surgery Certification, American Board of Cosmetic Surgery Certification, and American Board of Oral Maxillofacial Surgery Certification. I assumed that if the cosmetic surgeon couldn't do what I needed and wanted cosmetically, the medical doctor would kindly refer me to who he thought could do what I wanted and needed cosmetically. I discovered that the medical doctor I was dealing with had other cosmetic plans for me, which I found out later.

I never expected to be dealing with a professional predator who would set me up to be deceived prior to surgery. I never expected to be dealing with a professional con artist who would force major cosmetic changes to my nose and ears that were absolutely undeserved, positively inappropriate, and unacceptable to say the least. I would like to save the reader any similar painful cosmetic misery and malicious cosmetic failures, which are destructive to a person's mental and emotional health.

The actions of Dr. Cutter toward me were clearly below the standard of care by the nonrecognized cosmetic surgeon. I found out postsurgery that of the twenty-four boards of the American Board of Medical Specialties, Dr. Cutter was not listed on any one of them. The cosmetic results became a horrifying nightmare that I have endured ever since my surgery date in the nineties.

I was left in mental darkness for years as to the actual truth of my cosmetic deviations. The cosmetic results were more than scary for me. Dr. Cutter had done irreparable damage to my nose and ears. My cosmetic results ended up being painfully destructive in nature and in scope to my self-image and self-esteem. The adverse cosmetic changes were devastating and destructive to my unique facial features designed by my Creator, Jesus Christ.

My physical characteristics were designed to carefully reflect and mold God-given character in me. The painful cosmetic changes had the opposite effect upon my personality. My unique physical characteristics, created to exemplify my Creator's wonderful craftsmanship, were now agonizingly abnormal in appearance.

My faith in God has sustained me during difficult days, weeks, months, and years. My faith in God has sustained me during many hours of suffering in silence as normal-looking people kept doing the everyday things that they enjoy. I was clearly victimized by the nonrecognized cosmetic surgeon, but I continued to believe in God and I have hope for a better future. I continue to see the good in people, even though I know that I was positively victimized by a cosmetic predator who should have absolutely never touched my facial features with his cosmetic knife when he knew full well that he didn't have the specialized training in the nose and ears as an American Board Plastic Surgeon.

Postsurgery I asked my coworker Denise to call up and ask what Dr. Cutter's qualifications were. Denise didn't do exactly what I had requested for her to do. Instead, she identified herself to Dr. Cutter's receptionist, who answered her phone call, by using her middle name, April. She inquired of Dr. Cutter's receptionist that if she wanted to have surgery on her nose, she would want someone board-certified. The receptionist at first stated that there are a lot of boards out there. She then handed the phone to Dr. Cutter. Dr. Cutter shared with Denise thinking he was talking to a potential cosmetic patient named April that if she wanted a board-certified doctor, she would want Dr. Joseph Finney, MD, ABPS, in Champus. I had the opportunity to meet Dr. Finney one day after having another corrective revision change under my chin area by Dr. Raymond Rockwell.

Dr. Cutter won me over with Mr. Hyde, and he cut me up like Dr. Jekyll. Although Dr. Cutter took an irresistible cosmetic gamble on my facial features, he would find that my resilience to life's expectancies were not quickly forthcoming. God was still my life-sustaining source, but now I had persistent negative memories concerning Dr. Cutter.

When I was out walking one day with my wife, Lorena, I heard a man who had observed me as I walked by say, "Scary."

For me, it was another sad commentary, confirmation, and painful reminder of what Dr. Cutter had cosmetically done to me. I recognize that Dr. Cutter decided to tear down my cosmetic blueprint and rebuild it with something that would not be recognizable by me and the general public as something beautiful and normal looking in appearance. I want everyone to know that my cosmetic results regarding my facial features were not caused as a result of my own incessant pursuit of just any medical surgeon willingly eager and cosmetically able to perform surgical procedures regardless of precision expertise.

I knew that I was a cosmetic surgery victim, but I couldn't figure out what the boards were looking for to take disciplinary action or termination action against Dr. Cutter. Experientially I knew that the cosmetic violations were nothing short of cosmetic crimes. I never was successful in bringing a lawsuit against Dr. Cutter, and I continued to be reminded of the statute of limitations by paralegals and attorneys whenever I sought out legal help. Postsurgery, after I had met with an attorney within a two-year time frame to find out if I could bring a lawsuit against Dr. Cutter, the attorney couldn't really see that I had a case to pursue legal action against the doctor. I know for a solid absolute fact that the attorney caused me to miss out on bringing a lawsuit against the psycho doctor I had encountered. I chose to persist in pursuing a verdict, judgment, and ruling by the medical and dental boards that the medical doctor is licensed with. I felt that I needed closure concerning what I had endured at the hands of the cosmetic surgeon.

I had a good recollection of events that led up to my cosmetic and financial piracy, but I had difficulty psychologically putting my mental finger exactly on when and where the crime occurred. To make my points as hard-hitting as possible, I continued to utilize numerous illustrations of what I could remember had happened to me and the way I perceived the cosmetic violator. I discovered that for years, I wasn't able to precisely pinpoint the exact moment the crimes had taken place. I would need more time to get it exactly right.

I was let down by the legislators, the investigator unit, and the courts, which initially made the ruling regarding the statute of limitations in the state of Washington. I was let down by the attorney representing the legal system, who didn't recognize that I might possibly have significantly more time to prepare for a lawsuit against Dr. Cutter. I have learned that should a patient experience a loss of memory surrounding the medical malpractice event, he or she is then given an additional year to bring a lawsuit against a medical doctor, beyond the three-year statute of limitations. I experienced difficulty retrieving specific detailed memories after my dark encounter with Dr. Cutter. I was not able to fully figure things with precision and clarity exactly how Dr. Cutter had been successful at pulling off his cosmetic heist against me at this point in time. I came to realize that I was let down by the medical and dental boards, which did absolutely nothing to take legal action or bring disciplinary action against the medical doctor who had cut me up, except in one isolated case.

Dr. Cutter has ten complaints against him regarding his medical board status that I am aware of. All of them have been closed by his medical board. He has six closed complaints regarding his dental board status. Of the sixteen complaints, I discovered that the dental board brought disciplinary action against Dr. Cutter only one time for negligence. A liposuction patient died under his care due to his professional negligence.

I know that the laws need to be changed to allow the medical boards to have a criminal investigation team in each medical and dental board with strict enforcement powers. There must be strict enforcement against medical doctors violating the doctor-patient trust. The laws need to be changed so that, should a cosmetic consumer cry foul play at the hands of a medical doctor to the medical or dental boards, there would be an immediate, aggressive investigation by the criminal department. There would not be any delays by the medical board nor dental board to wait for years so that the patient can have adequate time to spiritually, mentally, and emotionally thaw out to have some semblance of internal equilibrium to completely figure out everything that happened to him or her. Should the legislators, judges, and medical and dental boards recognize this needed and required standard-of-care safeguard to protect the consumer, it could help to deter any medical doctor from thinking that his or her medical license and good standing are totally protected by the laws he or she is supposed to abide by. This would help to ensure against any medical doctor feeling narcissistic, powerful, and invincible concerning the medical, dental, and cosmetic consumer who comes under his or her care.

I learned the hard way from firsthand experience that there are predators in the medical field. Dr. Cutter's professional move to apprehend my cosmetic and financial business was completely unacceptable, destructive, and devastating to my person and mental health. I believe that Dr. Cutter was a blight on my life and he has become a blight on the life of other clients that he practiced on to improve his cosmetic skills.

I wish I had earnestly requested my coworker Denise, who provided a ride for me to and from surgery, never leave my side until my surgery was completely over with. By taking this added step of necessary protection, I might have been spared the malicious victimization by Dr. Cutter. I now wish that I had done my homework before coming in to see Dr. Cutter, which would have spared me needless suffering. This move became a huge, costly mistake for me. I was still asking questions of Dr. Cutter on the day of surgery when he made a bold move to aggressively move me into his presurgery, dimly lit room. I, like multitudes of others, wanted to trust a medical "expert," but I had the trust factor totally stripped from my life. Dr. Cutter became an ominous cosmetic nightmare of the worst kind for me.

I am persuaded that Dr. Cutter had to have seen himself as a bona fide cosmetic predator. No cosmetic surgeon would have used the malicious tactics that Dr. Cutter utilized on an unsuspecting patient like me unless he fully knew how to exploit the system that the medical boards operate under to increase his professional advantage. My friend Tommy Ray, who used to work the casinos in Las Vegas, Nevada, told me that he saw himself as a predator and he saw everyone else as his victims when they were sitting at the card tables. I assumed that Dr. Cutter had the good trust of the medical board and the good character to rightly inform me during our initial consultation of everything that he could or couldn't do cosmetically. Dr. Cutter told me, "I see ten different things wrong with your nose" and "How about this?" with a click on his computer mouse during our initial consultation. During our second consultation, Dr. Cutter stated, "I'm a perfectionist". Postsurgery, Dr. Cutter communicated to me, "It's what the other doctors did," after he messed up my nose and ears, which caused me to think that I had been dealing with a self-centered, ruthless, and abusive cosmetic surgeon.

I absolutely know for a 100 percent fact that my individual complaint case against Dr. Cutter has not been properly investigated by the medical review board or by the investigator unit. I am persuaded for a 100 percent fact that there should have been a criminal investigation called for by the investigator unit and the medical review board. But it never happened. Bumbling detective Colombo would have persisted until the case was 100 percent solved no matter how long it took.

My case has been put into limbo status. Although I have repeatedly requested a reconsideration for a new hearing by the medical review board, my case has continued to remain closed. I hope to change that situation one day. If I can do so, I finally might find closure to Dr. Cutter's criminal assault on my mind, which produced difficulties for me in retrieving memories postsurgery, and the cosmetic actions taken against me unmercifully back on the day of my surgeries. The inactions of the medical review board in completely not informing me of my rights effectively denied my constitutional rights as a patient. I needed help by a representative sent out by the medical review board and the investigator unit to help prepare the paperwork to pursue criminal charges against Dr. Cutter and rightly evaluate the cosmetic damages caused by a cosmetic predator, terrorist, and thug.

I contacted Robin at a referral service for cosmetic surgeons. I was told that cosmetic and plastic surgery are basically the same. I had heard similar statements in the past.

I shared with Robin that the cosmetic surgeon that I went to see was Outpatient Board Certified, and had listed himself in his full page ad in the yellow pages as American Board of Cosmetic Surgery and also American Board of Oral and Maxillofacial Surgery certified. I did not know how these so-called boards not recognized by the ABMS and the ABPS had qualified Dr. Cutter to do additional cutting on a multiple surgery patient like myself. The doctor's latter certification above meant that he was specialized in dentistry. None of his board statuses was as a plastic board-certified surgeon.

I informed Robin that I wasn't satisfied with the results. Robin went on to explain to me that, "The difference is the board certification of the doctor."

I inquired of Robin whether she might know about a doctor having a secondary in plastic surgery and a general in cosmetic surgery. She had no idea what all that meant. Robin told me that, "Nothing else really matters; it's the board certification."

She said, "If you want a specialist in plastic surgery, you must find a doctor, use a doctor who is certified by the American Board of Plastic Surgery. There is nothing equal to that."

Robin explained to me that, "The American Board of Medical Specialties is the board that oversees the subspecialty boards. They're like the top one that's going to oversee the boards. There is only one that is governed by them, and it's the American Board of Plastic Surgery."

Robin recognizes that the general public is much more informed than they were ten years ago. She also recognizes that people still need to do their research because some people are still not aware of the differences between the board-certified plastic surgeons and the nonrecognized-board medical doctors. This is where the horror stories come from: people going to doctors who are not specialists in that field of specialized training.

I inquired why a doctor who is not a specialist in that particular field would end up doing surgery on somebody, other than for the money. Robin recognized that it is about the money. Robin told me, "We don't have laws that control that."

I stated, "It has to start from the legislation and the courts if we're going to see a change."

Robin agreed with me.

"Otherwise, people are going down a precarious road," I said.

Robin affirmed that the medical boards have to make that change, which I understood to be a change in policy, which means that only certified American Board Plastic Surgeons, ABPS, and certified American Board Medical Specialists, ABMS, will be allowed to do any additional cosmetic or reconstruction work on a multisurgery patient. Furthermore, that no nonrecognized board medical doctors or nonrecognized board dentists or any other medical providers will be permitted to do additional cosmetic surgical cutting on a multisurgery patient, no matter how good or qualified they may think they are because of their years in practice.

Robin thinks that it is amazing that we don't have laws that govern this medical dilemma. She shared with me that some doctors take a weekend class to learn how to do a procedure, and they can go and do it. According to Robin, that's why it is so important to make sure you are dealing with a specialist.

I asked Robin if she knew of any book out there that she might recommend to the average cosmetic consumer who wants to make sure that he or she finds the right surgeon who can do precisely and exactly what he or she is asking for. Robin said, "No, there are no books for that. You just need to meet with the doctor. You start with the certification, and you go from there. You want to look at the before and after photos of previous patients. A reputable doctor will tell you if he can do what you're asking. If you've had a rhinoplasty and now you want a revisionary type surgery, he will be honest with you and tell you whether he can meet those expectations."

I inquired of Robin, "Other than just asking the doctor, how would you be able to know if they have gone for that weekend training?"

Robin said, "You want to make sure they are certified by the American Board of Plastic Surgery, that they are a specialist in that field."

Robin highly recommended a double-board plastic surgeon who had a good reputation for me to go to for my revision surgery.

I thanked Robin for talking with me on the phone. I never told Robin that the double-board plastic surgeon that she referred me to was Dr. James Evans, who performed my second rhinoplasty. I thought Dr. Evans did a pretty good job on my nose, but the surgery left the left side nostril somewhat higher positioned than my right-side nostril because of the missing cartilage.

It became an extremely scary situation when Dr. Cutter decided to take it upon himself to skip the subtle revisionary work that I was asking for. He simply tore down the previous doctor's work and rebuilt the nose in a higher-elevated position, which I was not wanting or needing cosmetically. Dr. Cutter also raised the right nostril to match my raised left nostril, totally against my cosmetic blueprint.

I recognize that Dr. Cutter has done some excellent cosmetic work, as told to me by a woman who works for a plastic surgeon in Champus. I also was informed by another woman, who works for a cosmetic surgeon, that the difference between plastic surgeons and cosmetic surgeons is that the plastic surgeon deals more with reconstruction surgery while the cosmetic surgeon primarily does cosmetic surgery to enhance a patient's physical beauty.

I contacted the Medical Quality Assurance Commission to inquire about Dr. Cutter's complaint status. I was informed that one patient had died under his care. The representative informed me that there was another patient complaint that ended in injury or death. The representative could not disclose to me the exact status of the other victimized patient. My position regarding my triple play surgeries and being victimized is that I curse the day that Dr. Cutter received his license to practice cosmetic surgeries.

I know that Dr. Cutter was delusional, with grandiose expectations that his nonrecognized-board status could possibly produce fantasy cosmetic results for me. Had I been a first-time patient of Dr. Cutter, my cosmetic results might have been different, with more positive consequences, even with his nonspecialized training in the nose and ears; but since I was a multiple cosmetic patient, I didn't need the mental trickery or thuggery forced on me by Dr. Cutter's manic tendencies. Keep in mind that the thought that my postsurgery cosmetic results might have been more to my liking as a potential first-time patient of Dr. Cutter's is merely speculative in scope relative to his noncertified board status with the ABMS and ABPS. I am persuaded that Dr. Cutter may have been on cocaine the day of surgery. Dr. Cutter had to have turned off the analytical center of his brain or he had to have a seared conscience for him to have successfully carried out such a malicious, sinister attack on me.

In my mind, only a real predator would have committed such a heinous cosmetic and financial heist against an innocent cosmetic consumer. I would like to save the reader the victimization that I have painfully endured all because I made some crucial assumptions that turned out to be major mistakes for myself.

Dr. Cutter's delusional thinking to act out his nonrecognized-board certification for the nose and ears on me was purely motivated by his own power and greed. Dr. Cutter had to have concluded that it was perfectly permissible to surgically do some additional cutting on a multiple surgery patient from the power base of his Outpatient Board Certification, American Board of Cosmetic Surgery, and his Oral Maxiallofacial Board certification status rather than from the proper certification of the American Board of Plastic Surgery. Had the medical board and dental boards rightly adopted and enacted a stiff law with hard-hitting penalties for any medical doctor violating a rule of performing surgeries on any multiple-surgery patient without being a qualified American Board Plastic Surgeon, such doctors would be immediately subject to termination. I would not have been mentally, emotionally, and cosmetically violated by Dr. Cutter.

The medical and dental review boards must wake up and smell the cosmetic coffee. They must open their eyes to objectively see that they cannot continue in the business of sufficiently safeguarding any unsuspecting consumer without taking on a criminal enforcement team.

Dr. Cutter would not be hiding behind his medical licensing board had there been a criminal enforcement team ready to take action provided any patient called out foul play by a medical doctor. Dr. Cutter would have been rooted out and prevented from ever practicing his medical and dental surgical procedures in Victimized, USA, ever again.

Dr. Cutter's delusional thinking, motivated by greed and power, would get cleared up, deleted, and eliminated in a hurry. Dr. Cutter's delusional thinking had opened the doors in his mind to erroneously think that there are a lot of boards out there. Dr. Cutter's thinking had infected his receptionist's thinking, as stated to Denise, my coworker, over the phone postsurgery.

If we were living in a perfect world, where every surgical procedure would produce 100 percent perfect results, I could agree to permit every medical doctor to perform multiple-surgery cosmetic procedures on any unsuspecting consumer any time and in whatever manner the medical surgeon deemed necessary, acceptable, and appropriate. If we were living in a totally accepting world, I could agree to allow medical malpractice crimes and abuses to continue in Victimized, USA. If ugly were in and beauty were out, I could agree to permit any cosmetic surgeons to carve and cut at will on any unsuspecting consumer because it wouldn't matter what a medical doctor surgically did. The results would always be in the doctor's favor, regardless of his needing to be a specialist in the field that you desired change for, in other words, certified by the ABMS or ABPS. We could allow the power-hungry, abusive, and greedy surgeons to make all the money that they wanted to without any medical restrictions and financial caps. But we are *not* living in a perfect world nor a totally accepting world. That's why we must shut down, stop at all costs, and eliminate all the Dr. Cutters of Victimized, USA, and Victimized, World. "And stop making excuses for them," as Bud would say.

I came to the powerful realization that certain medical doctors believe that they are masters of their own cosmetic universe and we, as their unsuspecting cosmetic consumers, are puppets in their cosmetic world. As puppets, we are forced to go along with their cosmetic agenda and accept the cosmetic results, however troubling, chaotic, and painfully devastating. As puppets, we are forced to deal with the painful cosmetic consequences and all the mental and emotional issues relative to these abnormal cosmetic changes.

I was seriously hurt by Dr. Cutter, and I was not willing to accept the cosmetic violations, deviations, and forced abnormal changes to my nose and ears willingly. I was going to fight back against my abductor by complaining to the licensing medical board and lawmakers. I was not going to be Dr. Cutter's puppet and foolishly accept his devious trickery and thuggery without objecting to these troubling changes. I objected to Dr. Cutter and to the medical board and to the legislators in Victimized, USA.

Since nothing has been done regarding Dr. Cutter's termination nor have they brought disciplinary action against him, if it were left up to me, I would shut down the entire medical board system at the MQAC and the Quality of Health Operation Commission in Olympia until Dr. Cutter was fired and had his board licensing suspended so he could never practice under his medical and dental board until he confessed to his cosmetic crimes and abuses against me. I have become dead serious and determined as a survivor of heinous crimes committed against me by the iron will of Dr. Cutter, and yet the iron will of justice has not been applied to him and to his board license status by the medical board, MQAC, or the dental board under the DQA Commission. From my perspective of being unjustly victimized by an uncaring medical doctor, it was not out of the question for me to think that the entire quality of health operation should be shut down until true justice prevailed against Dr. Cutter.

I was listening to a guest on Michael Medved's "nationally syndicated radio show broadcast locally on AM 770" between one and two o'clock one afternoon on my way to work, as I regularly would. Unfortunately for me, I never heard the name of Michael's guest, who happened to be talking about how politicians see the rest of us nonpoliticians as puppets of their universe. As I listened to Michael's guest share his incredible insight with the listening audience, his words caught my attention, and I in turn made the powerful connection to medical doctors like Dr. Cutter and others who are driven by self-interests as gods of their own world. It became crystal clear to me that medical doctors, like politicians, then force their subjects to go along with their self-interests, agendas, and greedy pursuits, to follow the way they see things in their own universe and the world they live in.

Being the masters of the Jewish people, the Nazi SS officers saw themselves as gods, who literally held the power of life and death over their Jewish slaves. It didn't matter how heinous and sinister their acts of mistreatment against their Jewish subjects were. Their delusional thinking empowered these SS officers to commit horrible atrocities against the Jewish captives because they were masters of their universe and they believed that the will of their fuehrer, Adolf Hitler, their leader, would last for a thousand years.

In like manner, Dr. Cutter's delusional thinking led him to believe that his cosmetic will forced on my facial features would last me the rest of my natural life. Instead, the cosmetic changes became my worst nightmare, which I still have to deal with today. Dr. Cutter had already hurt another man who felt like he had been butchered by him, and then he was willing to cosmetically violate me on top of that. Can Dr. Cutter's delusional thinking get any more obvious to the medical board, investigator unit, and legislators?

All legal authorities mentioned above must wake up to the atrocities being committed under their questionable seeing eyes of mental and health protection. Unsuspecting consumers, real people, are being victimized, abused, and hurt by real medical doctors.

I have come to the inevitable conclusion that Dr. Cutter had delusional thinking that led him to believe that his cosmetic surgical knife was quicker than my mind could perceive and faster than I could move my nose and ears out of his cosmetic way. You've heard the old saying, "The hand is quicker than the eye."

The evidence, based upon the facts of my experiences under Dr. Cutter's medical board professional care, has clearly shown that I was victimized by a medical doctor who knew that he did not have American Board of Plastic Surgery Certified training to qualify him as a specialist in the nose and ears, and yet Dr. Cutter played me for a fool who didn't have a brain in my head to rightly discern and properly evaluate exactly what happened to me pre- and postsurgery.

Dr. Cutter quickly forged ahead, making cosmetic changes that were scary, cruel, and painfully devastating to my nose and ears. Dr. Cutter knew that he deviously hurt me when he deceptively introduced mind-altering, hypnotic tactics and a chemical process or extreme form of radiation that would destroy my sense of discernment. By what I experienced postsurgery, having blankness and blackness on my memory bank with mental tension, I would testify that Dr. Cutter had to have utilized either a chemical process or a form of radiation that caused me to have mental paralysis or neutralization to prohibit me from retrieving detailed memory information of what led up to my surgeries, and prevent my mind from operating or functioning in a normal manner. This was Dr. Cutter's attempt to destroy my powerful memory, and it indicates just how spiritually sick Dr. Cutter truly is to stoop to criminal actions against me. Such actions clearly demonstrate just how cruel, criminal, and inhumane Dr. Cutter is as a medical doctor that he would victimize me for professional gain and personal profit.

It took a long process for me to figure out exactly what Dr. Cutter had mentally and cosmetically done to me. I wanted to be fair in my personal judgment of Dr. Cutter, and I wanted to be honestly accurate in my mental evaluation as to what I had experienced at the hands of Dr. Cutter. I do believe that Dr. Cutter acted alone in the mental trickery and thuggery he utilized on me; he wanted to use me to make the medical board believe that his nonrecognized-board status was just as qualified as an American Board of Plastic Surgery surgeon, which would keep the surgical doors open for other nonrecognized-board medical doctors to continue performing surgeries that they are not qualified to perform on unsuspecting consumers.

Going by what I have experienced at the surgical hands of Dr. Cutter, I know that Dr. Cutter used me as a sheep led to surgical slaughter for the love of filthy lucre and also to keep the surgical doors open for his nonrecognized-board certification status. In Dr. Cutter's mind, he had to have known that there was a lot at stake should I wake up and report that the medical board have another charlatan that they have to reel in.

I see these kinds of medical doctors as brute beasts who are willing to surgically carve up an unsuspecting consumer after mentally stunning him, which they know will leave that patient in a mental fog for years. These medical doctors are extremely afraid that their nonrecognized-board membership will be exposed as being a made-up board by certain medical doctors. They erroneously and delusively think that it would be a lot better for all of the nonrecognized medical doctors to continue performing cosmetic procedures on gullible patients, knowing that because of their ignorance of the many past practice-damaged patients, the percentages are on the side of these loose cannon medical doctors. These particular practitioners fear having their certifications yanked and their medical board status restricted from performing multiple surgical procedures on unsuspecting consumers.

The Medical Quality Assurance Commission needs to change its medical policies to state that positively no board-certification medical doctor other than one with an American Board of Plastic Surgery Certification will ever be allowed to perform or conduct surgeries on a multiple-surgery patient. If the legislators, medical and dental review boards, judges, and courts of Victimized, USA, don't enact new laws to put an immediate stop to the victimization, I recognize that there are many more delusional-thinking predators eagerly waiting to begin surgical procedures on innocent, unsuspecting cosmetic consumers. We will see many more complaints of medical malpractice crimes and abuses by certain medical doctors intoxicated with power, greed, and self-interests if these laws are not implemented by the above powers. They need to pull together to enact and enforce stiff laws and high penalties to discourage predators from exploiting the trusting and unsuspecting public.

I am not opposed to plastic and cosmetic surgery practice as a physical enhancement business operation. I am also not against the doctors who have diligently earned each of their board certification statuses by being certified by the American Board of Cosmetic Surgery, the American Board of Oral Maxillofacial Surgery, or listing themselves as Board-Certified with nothing added under the ad. It could read: Certified Outpatient Surgery Center, followed by the office address. The above-mentioned are legitimate boards with unique specialization in their own right. These boards are recognized by their own membership, and they would definitely fall into the category of "There are a lot of boards out there," as stated by Dr. Cutter's receptionist. Carrie Barkley (the new deputy executive director at the MQAC) inquired if I would like to talk to a medical doctor on hand at the MQAC in Olympia. The medical doctor stated to me over the phone the exact same thing Dr. Cutter's receptionist had said: "There are a lot of boards out there."

Keep in mind that the above boards are not recognized by the American Board of Plastic Surgery and by the American Board of Medical Specialties. I strongly recommend that all doctors and the medical and dental commissions governing each medical doctor's licensing come to recognize their shortcomings and limitations in regard to cosmetic specifications on unsuspecting multiple-surgery patients. The medical and cosmetic surgery procedure policies must be changed now, or there will continue to be a steady stream of physical, emotional, and mental devastation that is foreseeable, avoidable, and needless. The painful and physically devastating consequences on unsuspecting real people are too scary to contemplate.

I unfortunately will not have the opportunity to take Dr. Cutter to court over his cosmetic and financial crimes committed against me due to the fact that the statute of limitations has run out for me. My compelling case presented in *The Ultimate Violation* will now be heard by the whole wide world to render its verdict against the cruel victimization I experienced at the surgical hands of Thadeaus Damon Cutter, DDS, MD. I never had the chance to explain the crimes committed against me before a judge and jury in the William County Courthouse in downtown Union. I am asking for an occasion to share the honest truth and present the facts based on actual experience to support my story of how I was cosmetically and financially victimized in Union by a nonrecognized cosmetic surgeon. I request that the reader render an honest intellectual judgment giving your verdict against my victimization, which took place in our great country of the United States of America. I am encouraged to think that my case of victimization could help set a precedent to bring about a belated but needful change in the current medical policies to abolish all forms of medical malpractice and medical negligence in the United States and throughout the world.

I know for a 100 percent fact that Dr. Cutter took full advantage of this official discrepancy in the lack of policy matters by the Medical Quality Assurance Commission and exploited me in every way possible for his own self-interests at my expense. I was and am a real person encountering a medical doctor who had delusional and mental fantasies of grandiose cosmetic achievements that he was not specialized in. I recognize for a 100 percent fact that Dr. Cutter completely misinterpreted my cosmetic interests for my nose and ears, and totally misunderstood what I cosmetically wanted, needed, and expected. I know that I have been misunderstood by a good number of my carrier professional colleagues and by the general public. I have come to realize that Dr. Cutter utilized a psychological blitzkrieg of bamboozlement to my mental perception to advance his cosmetic agenda against me. I know for a 100 percent fact that the medical licensing board and the chief investigator along with the investigator unit were completely fooled and deceived by Dr. Cutter's actions against me. I can understand Dr. Cutter's actions in light of Jon Meacham's quote in *Newsweek* of December 29, 2008/January 5, 2009: "From Plato forward, philosophers have struggled to define power, which is at heart the capacity to bend reality to your will." According to my friend Bud, "This quote could also apply toward people's perception of reality, which can and has been bent to their detriment by the media and social planners."

I became another hurt victim in the long history seen in the abuse of power at the surgical hands of a predator disguised as a specialist in dentistry, DDS. I was totally unable to prevent the cosmetic surgeon from exploiting my cosmetic and financial business on that unfortunate day of surgery. If the legislators, medical board, dental board, judges, and courts of the United States of America do absolutely nothing to create and enact laws to prevent medical malpractice crimes and abuses, then there are scores of medical doctors who are waiting in the ranks of the medical boards who will continue to victimize other unsuspecting consumers.

When I received my first letter from an insurance company concerning my injuries postsurgery with Dr. Cutter, I didn't know what to do with it at first. The insurance company provides insurance claims for hospitals and doctors, I was told. After some consideration, I sent back the letter providing my submitted information regarding what I should be compensated for. My request for financial compensation was denied by the insurance company. Postsurgery I had shared my unhappiness with Dr. Cutter's secretary over the phone, and she told me that I needed to talk to Dr. Cutter. I was daily right in the middle of dealing with a constant state of mental barriers and blockades from Dr. Cutter's stunning mental whammy against my mind, along with the physical cosmetic devastation I was experiencing and negative reactions from a lot of the general public. I also talked to Francis Fergeson, who deals with medical malpractice in the Lone Star state of Texas.

When I was talking with Francis and inquiring if I had any legal recourse to pursue a lawsuit against Dr. Cutter, it became obvious to me that Francis had a good understanding of my predicament regarding the three-year statute of limitations that exists in Washington state. Francis mentioned that in the state of Texas, they have a two-year statute of limitations.

I knew from personal experience what Francis was talking about when she stated, "When a patient begins to thaw out," referring to the mental trauma and shock a stunned patient goes through during a medical malpractice experience. Any medical doctor that has to resort to committing medical malpractice by storming the brain with dirty mental hypnotic neutralization tactics should be banned from ever performing cosmetic surgeries on another potential victim and stripped from his or her medical license outright.

My sister Marlie informed me of a conversation she had with an attorney Paul Davis in Clover Valley. Paul told Marlie that there will be forty thousand fewer doctors by the year 2020. Paul went on to explain to Marlie the reason for the shortage in medical doctors will be due to the statistics of medical malpractice suits and fewer doctors choosing to go into the medical field.

What I experienced at the hands of a medical doctor willing to exploit and utterly take advantage of me mentally, cosmetically, and financially, when he fully knew that he lacked the cosmetic and reconstruction expertise of a qualified Certified American Board of Plastic Surgeon, is in my perspective 100 percent evil.

When power trippers and delusional-thinking medical doctors are willing to commit cosmetic and financial crimes against innocent, unsuspecting consumers, it's high time to pull the plug on their licensing to practice cosmetic surgery before they have another opportunity to hurt, abuse, and victimize another unsuspecting patient. My victimization was purely about Dr. Cutter's show, and positively not about my personal cosmetic interests.

I would like for the reader to keep in mind that there are psychotic predators in the medical fields with smiling faces waiting for you to enter their cosmetic psycho web. These medical predators haven't had the specialized training in specific body areas as have members of the twenty-four boards of medical specialties. These medical doctors may have delusional thinking of possibly using you to add to their cosmetic statistics and financial gain to prove to themselves that they can deceive you and fool the medical board regarding "There are a lot of medical boards out there." I have come to recognize that these medical doctors are slackers and predators; they are delusional, psychotic, and power-tripping thinkers who are ready and willing to victimize unsuspecting consumers for personal profit and professional gain. They are not about to be stopped until the medical board recognize that these delusional-thinking power trippers, operating as medical doctors, are on a runaway train with your cosmetic and financial business at stake. I recognize that they must be stopped in their tracks immediately with the stroke of a pen by the legislators in Olympia and by the US Congress through enacting laws that have real teeth to them.

I have come to the realization that the object of these nonrecognized-board certified doctors is to wait to catch the unsuspecting consumer mentally off guard on the very day of surgery. They purposely play along with the unsuspecting patient, who may be in the process of attempting to explain in detail to the cosmetic surgeon exactly what he or she cosmetically wants, needs, and expects regarding results and outcome.

The cosmetic surgeon then says something like, "Well, I better go about building up the bridge" as he mentally pushes you over into the unconscious realm so that you are incapable of reversing your cosmetic tracks and quickly making your escape out of the consultation room before going into his presurgery, dimly lit room, where the medical doctor now can tell and show you his cosmetic agenda. You are now at the mercy of the malicious medical doctor who has the mind-set that he cares more about capturing your cosmetic and financial business than he cares about your self-interests.

When Dr. Cutter said, "Well, I better go about building up the bridge," I now know that that was his call for me to go into a prehypnotic altered state of mind. I remember wondering why Dr. Cutter hadn't told me during our initial consultation that he planned on building up the bridge of my nose, which I clearly didn't want, need, nor expect cosmetically. I wasn't interested at all in having my nose bridge built up. As I thought on this situation following the doctor into a dark room, my mind suddenly went blank.

I was powerless to stop Dr. Cutter's reverse psychological mind control tactics of taking charge of my cosmetic destiny, which he was utilizing against me. Dr. Cutter was not playing fair with me every step of the way. I had been caught in and swallowed up by Dr. Cutter's psychoheresy web, meaning "psychological or mind deception tactics, which is the integration of mind-altering techniques and theories. It's like Christ-centered ministry versus problem-centered counseling. There is a world of difference," as my friend Bud put it. I found the mind deception techniques of Dr. Cutter was not a fun place to be, and the consequences are totally avoidable provided the Medical Quality Assurance Commission changes its governing policies restricting nonrecognized medical doctors from ever performing surgeries on multiple-surgery patients like myself.

At this juncture, Dr. Cutter had pushed me over mentally into the unconscious dimension, where he could program me subconsciously for his cosmetic agenda, which I didn't recognize postsurgery. Dr. Cutter knew what he was going to do to me, but I didn't know what Dr. Cutter was going to do to me. I have been able to slow down the process for the reader;

at the time, things kept on moving at a rather fast pace, which caught me mentally completely off guard. Dr. Cutter was not going to give me time to think it through nor time to mentally digest what Dr. Cutter was now ready to do to me. In fact, Dr. Cutter wasn't going to permit me the consideration of making a mental decision for or against what Dr. Cutter was now planning to cosmetically do to me in the unconscious realm.

I bear scars under both of my breasts giving testimony and providing evidence that Dr. Raymond Rockwell had to remove cartilage from my rib cage just to help lower my nose; Dr. Cutter had purposely raised my nose into an elevated place and repositioned it in an arrangement against my will that looks abnormal in appearance. That is scary.

By this time, you have unknowingly entered the doctor's mental and cosmetic playground, wherein the maze of postsurgery conscious and unconscious mental confusion has now blurred the mental lines as to exactly what has happened to you mentally, cosmetically, and financially. The psychotic, delusional, and power-tripper medical doctor has you exactly where he wants you to be. He knows that it may take years for you to figure out what has just happened to you at the hands of the nonrecognized medical doctor. How are you going to prove what has happened to you to the medical boards, an attorney, or the judicial courts of the land in Victimized, USA, *and* Victimized, World?

How long will it take to possibly know within yourself that you are mentally capable of explaining precisely what the psychotic, sociopathic, and delusional-thinking medical doctor has done to you? You feel that things have gotten turned around in your mind, and you feel violated by a medical doctor who shouldn't have touched your facial features in the first place. After explaining what you can mentally remember has happened to you to the people who you believe you can trust, whether you realize it or not, you are working your way through a depression, trauma, and psychological whammy that the subspecialty cosmetic medical doctor has dragged you into. You have been dragged into the maze of the web of psycho "deception techniques, that is, psychoheresy deception tactics. In fact, it is a self-esteem-centered religion," as my friend Bud, aka Brutus Knuckles, put it. The bottom line of exactly why any medical doctor would ever do something like what I went through is clearly for self-interests, greed, and power on the part of the medical doctor.

I have come to see Dr. Cutter as another pathetic coward, who was eagerly ready and willing to do some more cutting and rearranging on my nose and ears because he had not been and was not restricted by the medical boards to stop performing surgical procedures on multiple-surgery patients. The medical boards had not restricted Dr. Cutter from his mayhem against unsuspecting patients, although he knew within himself that he was not an American Board Certified Plastic Surgeon. Because Dr. Cutter had not been restricted by clear guidelines set down by the medical boards due to his lack of medical specialty training, I was cosmetically and financially ripped off by a cosmetic predator, violator, and terror intruder disguised as a medical doctor.

The tactics Dr. Cutter utilized against me, who was positively an unsuspecting, multiple-surgery cosmetic consumer, need to be exposed and eliminated to never be utilized on another unsuspecting patient in Victimized, USA, and Victimized, World. I thank God I was given an opportunity to tell my horrible cosmetic ordeal to save others the painful mental, emotional, and cosmetic misery I have personally experienced.

I have seen a Christian counselor on and off for years regarding my agonizing cosmetic ordeal at the hands of Dr. Cutter. I have also gone to see a professional psychologist, Willis M. Dunken, PhD, ABPP, who is certified by the American Board of Professional Psychology and the American Board of Psychological Hypnosis.

I wanted to see if the professional psychologist could recognize that I had been hypnotized by Dr. Cutter in his dimly lit, presurgery room. I gave psychologist Dunken a description of some of the things that I remembered experiencing on the day of surgery, when Dr. Cutter took charge of my cosmetic destiny.

Mr. Dunken told me, "By your description, I wouldn't know if you were hypnotized or not."

I know within myself by what has taken me years to figure out that Dr. Cutter did utilize some form of hypnosis and some form of radiation or chemical to cause memory loss for a long period of time as to what I had experienced. It took me eight to nine years to come to a complete understanding and fully know what happed to me with absolute certainty. My friend Tommy Ray, having served in Vietnam, believes that it was something chemical-related that Dr. Cutter utilized on me based on what I told him about the things that I experienced under Dr. Cutter's care. I recognize that Tommy is not an expert nor any type of an authority on the use of chemical or radiation per se. It was only just a thought that came to his mind when I shared with him what I had experienced postsurgery under Dr. Cutter's care.

Psychologist Dunken told me that if he used hypnosis on me to regress back in my mind, it would ruin my testimony in the courts, since the opposing attorney would argue that Dunken had influenced me to think such things. I told Mr. Dunken that I wasn't thinking of having him use hypnosis on me.

I know that I don't need to have a psychiatrist or a psychologist determine exactly what I underwent at the hands of Dr. Cutter. I know that Dr. Cutter was on a power trip to move out of his medical specialty, which is in dentistry, DDS, to want to take on a multiple-surgery patient like myself. To preserve his own ego and whatever conscience he might have, Dr. Cutter had to have been in an altered state of mind, such as a predator or a criminal mind-set, to do what he did to me. I know that Dr. Cutter had to have turned off his conscience or turned off the analytical center of his brain to commit his cosmetic and financial crime against me. I know beyond a shadow of a doubt that Dr. Cutter was too wrapped up in his self-interest pursuit of plundering my cosmetic and financial business to think clearly what consequences his actions would have on me.

I remember speaking to a woman who uses hypnotism in her therapy practice on patients in the Banner district in Union. I inquired if, as a consequence of utilizing hypnotism on a person, there is any residual blackness or blankness left on the memory bank of a patient. I recollect the female therapist saying, "Oh no, you have been watching too many late movies." She answered my quest for answers concerning what I had experienced postsurgery with Dr. Cutter. I was convinced beyond a shadow of a doubt that I had been victimized and that criminal actions were committed against me by what I had experienced at the cruel hands of Dr. Cutter pre- and postsurgery.

A man named Sid Advice, who works for the Medical Quality Assurance Commission, told me, "If it still bothers you, why don't you seek legal help?" From my perspective, I thought Sid's advice was poor advice to offer a patient continuously suffering from being victimized by a malicious predator. I realize that Sid didn't have a clue relative to everything I had been going through postsurgery. I had sought legal help from attorneys, but to no avail. I would have appreciated Sid, out of a sincere heart of understanding and care, showing me some respect and consideration concerning my desire of wanting to hear that the medical and dental boards decided to take disciplinary or termination action against Dr. Cutter. That never took place.

I would replace Sid Advice if I had the power to do so for his insensitive remarks to a cosmetic victim who was clearly victimized by Dr. Cutter. I would also shut down the Medical Quality Assurance Commission if I could until they instate new policies regarding nonrecognized cosmetic surgeons and tell Dr. Cutter to pack his cosmetic bags and hit the road for his ruinous actions against my nose and ears. I strongly know that the nonaction verdict by the medical review board against Dr. Cutter was pathetic, and I firmly believed that their lack of action would give Dr. Cutter the green light to continue hurting other unsuspecting patients. I called up and voiced my disappointment for their decision not to take any disciplinary action against Dr. Cutter. I needed a positive verdict by the board that I truly was victimized and that it was not a mere slip of Dr. Cutter's cosmetic knife that caused irreparable damages to my nose and ears.

I know that Dr. Cutter's actions against me were not an accident, but cosmetic and financial crimes. Dr. Cutter's actions against me were destructive to my total being, dignity, and character; they have consumed numerous hurtful, abusive, and wasted years in my life, which could have clearly been avoided by Dr. Cutter had he only told the truth up front during our initial consultation. Instead, Dr. Cutter chose to use me for his personal exploitation and professional gain, and as a result, I have painfully suffered throughout the years. I did not need Dr. Cutter's professional mental trickery and thuggery, which led to my cosmetic surgery, causing me irreparable damages to my nose and ears. Dr. Cutter's actions on the day of my surgeries were clearly not in my cosmetic and financial self-interests, to say the least. I want to repeat an earlier statement that I know to be 100 percent true: If any one of the medical board members had experienced what I have endured at the hands of Dr. Cutter, they would clearly say, "Truly this was a cosmetic and financial crime if there ever was one. Such actions committed against an unsuspecting patient like myself would be considered and classified as medical malpractice."

I have learned that the reason why the medical board hasn't closed the legal doors on nonrecognized cosmetic surgeons who have committed medical malpractice actions against unsuspecting patients is due to greed.

I had another talk with Robin regarding the reason why the medical boards throughout the land haven't intervened in this problem with unqualified medical doctors. I asked, "They're leaving the doors open to medical doctors who are not qualified to work on certain patients. Why haven't they come up with stricter laws concerning this serious situation?"

Robin answered me with, "That's a good question. I don't know why they haven't." She communicated that it would be a good question for a doctor to answer. Indeed, I want to know, "Why haven't the medical boards enforced strict guidelines on irresponsible doctors and surgeons committing irresponsible acts on their patients?"

I want to see complete and thorough action taken immediately by the US Congress, legislators throughout the land, courts and judges, and the medical and dental boards throughout our country to ensure more legal recourse for patients who have been done wrong. The cost of legal action on the part of the patient should be absorbed by the doctors committing the criminal actions of irresponsibility against the patients. That would be reinforced by the state.

I have discovered a lot of things postsurgery since I first encountered Dr. Cutter. The cosmetic deck was stacked against me from the outset of meeting Dr. Cutter during our initial consultation. I discovered that Dr. Cutter was not specialized in the nose and ears as an American Board of Plastic Surgery surgeon; I was searching for such qualifications when I first came in to see Dr. Cutter, as indicated by my postsurgery desired results notes.

I have realized that Dr. Cutter did his level best to tear down the previous doctor's work and rebuild my nose with a counterfeit substitute and imitation, having raised and repositioned my nose, causing it to appear abnormal in appearance. My nose and ears were altered with irreparable damages that I clearly didn't want, need, or expect.

I discovered that the statute of limitations was running out on me from ever pursuing a lawsuit against Dr. Cutter due to the medical board not informing me about all of my rights and the steps I should take to see justice served. The juries are not sympathetic toward injured, abused, and victimized multisurgery patients. Because of the above-mentioned facts, I know that there will be many more victimized, unsuspecting patients until the medical board stop pandering to delusional and power-tripper medical doctors with an insatiable desire for filthy lucre and their lust for greed, professional gain, and personal profit.

I know that Dr. Cutter was making some strong statements when he set out to victimize me. Dr. Cutter was making a powerful statement that you don't need to have all the extra training that the Certified American Board of Plastic Surgeons requires. He was stating that you can depend on mental trickery and thuggery as a delusional cosmetic slacker, and still produce positive cosmetic physical enhancements when operating on unsuspecting, multiple-surgery patients.

Dr. Cutter was clearly making a statement that he could do whatever he wanted to cosmetically do to me because the medical board have left the doors wide open for him to literally have his cosmetic way with patients, as many unsuspecting patients as he wants to, until they put a screeching halt on his insatiable appetite for power, greed, and personal self-interests.

He was making a statement, "I am going to have my way with Kurtess because he is a cosmetic simpleton since he was the one who came into my cosmetic practice and will accept my deranged cosmetic violations and deviations without detection because I have the power to do so without impunity and because I am smart enough not to repeat the same criminal action to get caught and come under the scrutiny of any medical review board because they are my puppets, too." Dr. Cutter knows that there are no stool pigeons who are on the medical review board acting as spies to report criminal wrongdoings to the police.

Medical doctors who are sinister predators look for weaknesses in the system, and they look for ways to exploit the unsuspecting patient to avoid detection of their criminal actions against the innocent victim. They criminally assault the brain of the unsuspecting patient so that they are left mentally short-circuited, impaired, and confused for years as to exactly what happened to them during surgery. If they complain negatively to the medical review board, they can end up looking like mentally deranged patients.

Dr. Cutter, like many other nonrecognized certified medical doctors, are not going to stop making additional cosmetic changes to unsuspecting patients since they haven't been caught or stopped in their conniving cosmetic tracks. Therefore they are permitted to repeat their delusional, deranged, manic, psychotic, sinister, sociopathic, and psychopathic actions against all the unsuspecting patients that they want to until the victimized patient fights back by reporting them to the medical board, investigator unit, and Better Business Bureau.

The medical board, MQAC, is then forced to put a stop to their criminal victimization by recognizing that these delusional-thinking medical doctors are setting a pattern of malicious cosmetic butchery that is totally below the standard of care as set forth by the health departments throughout our country and the Medical Quality Assurance Commission.

I want to alert the reader to the dangers that are in the medical and business community. I experienced a major pitfall that awaited my searching, questioning, and trusting patient attitude. I realize that trust in human relationships is important, but this does not mean having a blind trust. The same goes for a doctor-patient relationship. I was questioning while searching for the right cosmetic surgeon, and I never expected a medical doctor in a position of trust would betray my trust. I discovered the trust factor was violated by a medical doctor feigning to be a cosmetic specialist in the nose and ears, but in actuality he was a wolf in medical garb. In the understanding of Dr. Cutter, an unsuspecting patient used and abused is better than one walking away from his office and out of his dimly lit, presurgery room. How does the reader know if he has encountered a sinister predator disguised as a medical doctor, as I did?

The cosmetic surgeon stays close to you mentally to crowd your thinking. He doesn't want you to think long and hard about what he can and can't do cosmetically for you. This is an approach where you are allowed to come to your own short conclusions, and then he continues to work on your mind to keep you mentally starved and off balance to catch you completely off guard with his cosmetic scam, scheme, and heist. Once you think he has utilized his approach of allowing you to come to any type of positive cosmetic conclusions regarding your postsurgery desired results, he suddenly runs a reverse psychological whammy on you by telling you, "Well, I better go about building up the bridge." This may not be something that you wanted to have done in your specific and detailed cosmetic blueprint.

As I began to think about Dr. Cutter not telling me up front of his plans to build up the bridge of my nose, my mind went blank within one to two seconds as I followed the doctor into the darkened room. I remember I had bumped into Dr. Cutter directly after I entered the dark room, and my mind went suddenly blank. Dr. Cutter had succeeded at allowing me to come to my own initial conclusions that he was qualified to meet my cosmetic interests for my nose, ears, and chin, only to pull a psycho deception tactics whammy on me by informing me of his cosmetic agenda for my nose shortly before my mind went mentally blank, and shortly after I had anesthesia administered for my cosmetic surgeries. Dr. Cutter didn't tell me all of the plans he envisioned for me in specific detail because he knew that had he done so, I would have walked out of his office and consultation rooms and never come back.

Dr. Cutter instead wanted to use me for his own professional statistics, personal profit, and cosmetic agenda by purposefully waiting and withholding vital cosmetic information from me only to make up things postsurgery with poor excuses. By the time I had awakened to the fact that I had experienced cosmetic violations and major deviations to my nose and ears, it was too late. I already had my cosmetic and financial business under Dr. Cutter's control.

After subduing me mentally, Dr. Cutter was prepared to fill in the blanks postsurgery. Initially postsurgery, Dr. Cutter filled in one big blank by saying, "See it as a sculpture. I tore it down, beat it up, and built it back up." As I began to think about the words that Dr. Cutter had told me postsurgery, I began to question in my mind why Dr. Cutter hadn't informed me of his cosmetic plans up front. Never mind that I came to the realization that I felt used, abused, ripped off, and violated. Dr. Cutter was now ready to reveal to me the truth about the mask he had hidden behind in his fantasy thinking and the harsh reality that his patient was seriously hurt by telling me, "It didn't turn out as I had envisioned." He also said to me, "It's what the other doctors did."

I found that Dr. Cutter would frequently have his nursing consultant, who also was his photo technician, around during our postsurgery consultations to catch anything I might say should I proceed in pursuing a lawsuit against him. Dr. Cutter had his witness in place to protect him from any scrupulous character who might sue him for damages.

I am a victim of dirty cosmetics from my patient's perspective, and I know that it's true that Dr. Cutter didn't rightly interpret my cosmetic interests. Nonetheless, he was able to plunder my cosmetic and financial business before I was able to leave from his professional practice on the day of my surgeries.

I know that I was dealing with and was victimized by a cosmetic predator, a psychopathic and sociopathic cosmetic surgeon. I found that

Dr. Cutter was making up things postsurgery to me after apprehending my cosmetic and financial business. I have come to the inevitable conclusion that the object of these fantasy cosmetic predators is to keep you mentally starved and off balance so that they are then able to make up things postsurgery to cover their cosmetic fannies. Not informing you of every detailed cosmetic procedure up front is strong evidence that they lack the cosmetic specialization training that a Certified American Board Plastic Surgeon has. I want to warn the reader of medical predators who care more about gaining your cosmetic and financial business than care about you as an individual with specific, detailed cosmetic wants, needs, and expectations.

I discovered that Dr. Cutter's approach with me turned out to be a one-way professional and cosmetic street from Dr. Cutter to myself. I found that it positively wasn't the other way around. When I began to question Dr. Cutter approximately three months after my surgeries regarding my nose in front of my coworker Denise, Dr. Cutter acted like he was on a power trip toward me. When I came in for a postsurgery consultation with Dr. Cutter approximately six months after surgery without any witnesses around, he acted like a guilty, eccentric medical doctor who was having extreme difficulties handling any questions from me.

As related above, I questioned Dr. Cutter by saying, "What happened to my nose? It looks like a turtle nose."

Dr. Cutter immediately turned around, stood up, and began looking up at the wall. As he looked up at the wall with his back turned toward me, Dr. Cutter responded to my question and said, "If something could be done, we'd have to wait a year."

Dr. Cutter then stated, "I hope it will come down."

When Dr. Cutter finally turned around to sit down behind a desk in front of me, he looked at me and said, "It didn't turn out as I envisioned."

I responded to Dr. Cutter by saying, "My complaint is that it not only didn't turn out as I envisioned, but it also has to do with the way that you went about getting my business."

At first, Dr. Cutter just looked at me, and then he dropped his head as if he didn't want to deal with what he had done to me any longer. Dr. Cutter never responded to my last, poignant comments regarding the approach that he had taken with me.

The Ultimate Violation

I came to the realization that Dr. Cutter pushed his cosmetic agenda onto me because he needed to fool and deceive the medical board as well as the investigator unit of his mental trickery and thuggery. I came to the realization that what I had experienced at the hands of Dr. Cutter wasn't a surgical accident, but cosmetic and financial crimes of horrible, irreparable nose and ear damages, with postsurgery mental and emotional anguish, including long-term reflections on Dr. Cutter. I continuously reflected on the kind of medical doctor that I had encountered and how he had violated me mentally and cosmetically unnecessarily. I found myself reflecting on the events leading to his cosmetic crimes over and over for days and months, and throughout the years. I could feel and sense the psychological whammy in my mind clouding, preventing me from figuring out exactly what Dr. Cutter had done to me mentally and cosmetically.

Dr. Cutter's actions had caused the chemistry in my brain to be negatively impacted. I knew within myself that Dr. Cutter had committed a crime against me, but I found that it was hard to bring any convincing evidence to the medical board to either bring disciplinary action against him or especially to bring a verdict of termination against him. As far as I was concerned, if I was the chairman of the medical or dental board, I would have told Dr. Cutter to pack his cosmetic bags and hit the road. He would not be allowed to practice under his medical or dental board license once he received my verdict.

I have come to realize that Dr. Cutter now has twelve closed complaints against him under his medical board. My cosmetic debacle and series of complaint letters, which also included a series of requests for a criminal investigation, were placed under his medical board. He has six complaints against him under his dental board, and complaint number five ended in death. I am convinced that once a medical doctor is accused and convicted of a crime in one of his medical or dental board license categories or status, he or she should not be allowed to practice under another board membership or license.

I have come to realize that Dr. Cutter didn't allow me to have the freedom of thought to decide whether I would submit myself to hypnosis. Dr. Cutter just took over as a cosmetic shark without discussion and began cutting and carving on me like I was a piece of meat. Dr. Cutter aggressively took over and helped himself, doing some additional cutting on my nose and ears without my knowledge and consent. Dr. Cutter ruthlessly and maliciously began doing additional cutting on my facial features totally against my cosmetic wants, needs, expectations, and desired interests. These were all gradual realizations that I came to as the years ground unmercifully by.

I contacted the disclosure department at the Medical Quality Assurance Commission again to check up on Dr. Cutter's complaint status. I previously discovered that Dr. Cutter had ten complaints under his medical license, which were all closed except for one open complaint that was pending. This time when I inquired, his complaint status had changed from ten to twelve closed complaints. He had six closed complaints under his dental license and one open that was pending prior to my last check. He had one under his general anesthesia license that was open and pending.

I can only hope that Dr. Cutter and other predatory medical doctors are stopped from hurting victims in the course of their professional practice. Perhaps Dr. Cutter has modified his predatory actions on unsuspecting patients to comply with the policies of the medical board, dental board, and the commission's rules. Possibly his nonrecognized board status has caught the full attention of the medical board he is licensed with, and he has reached the maximum complaint status without drawing more scrutiny to the list of injured patients.

I realized that dealing with Dr. Cutter was like dealing with a cosmetic phantom. The day before my surgeries, my nose and ears were doing just fine; I wanted to have some cosmetic enhancements for them with subtle cosmetic changes. The day of my surgeries in the nineties, I was subjected to a malicious assault on my nose and ears by an unqualified cosmetic surgeon who was a greedy opportunist; he was an MD, DDS who didn't have specialty training in the nose and ears, which I wanted and needed. I understand now exactly why Dr. Cutter had to become sinisterly malicious with me: I wouldn't have stayed around had Dr. Cutter told me the truth. Dr. Cutter made his aggressive move to prevent me from mentally waking up to say, "I don't feel comfortable with your approach, and I would like to leave here now."

Dr. Cutter mentally desensitized me so that I became nonreactive to what Dr. Cutter was going to do to me cosmetically. I came to realize that Dr. Cutter impaired my mental perceptions so that I was rendered mentally ineffective at rightly discerning the doctor's actions, and his deceptive approach, which resulted in scary cosmetic violations and deviations and painful cosmetic irreparable damages.

I am convinced that I was cosmetically and financially victimized by Dr. Cutter. I know without any doubt that cosmetic and financial crimes were committed against me by Dr. Cutter. When I asked Dr. Raymond Rockwell if he considered the cosmetic work by Dr. Cutter a crime, Dr. Rockwell responded to me by telling me that if Dr. Cutter had left an orange peeling or a peanut shell inside of my nose, then he would have considered it a crime. I shared some of the things that Dr. Cutter had done to me on the day of surgery, but I know that Dr. Rockwell didn't experience what I had, with the horrible postsurgery consequences. I allowed Dr. Rockwell to share his professional opinion without trying to convince him otherwise.

When I inquired of Dr. Rockwell's professional opinion, I still hadn't been able to totally figure out everything conclusively regarding my victimization; I was still unable to pinpoint the exact moment the actual crimes had been committed against me by Dr. Cutter. When Dr. Cutter pushed me over into the unconscious realm, I had no partial or full understanding to be able to respond or react in a normal way to what Dr. Cutter was going to cosmetically do to me. I know that Dr. Raymond Rockwell is not a forensic or a cosmetic criminologist who could prove that I was victimized by Dr. Cutter.

Dr. Cutter knew what he was going to do cosmetically to his subdued patient, but I didn't know what Dr. Cutter was going to do to me cosmetically because I had no knowledge of Dr. Cutter's cosmetic agenda and plans on the day of my surgeries. I have come to realize that Dr. Cutter had reversed his cosmetic agenda on me without my knowledge and consent. Dr. Cutter reversed his cosmetic course after desensitizing my mind, which provides all the convincing evidence that he fully knew that he didn't have the specialization in the nose and ears that I was asking for in my desired postsurgery notes. Dr. Cutter was headstrong in wanting my cosmetic and financial business anyway. Therefore, the medical board need to come to a mutual decision and to a unanimous verdict that cosmetic and financial crimes were committed against me.

I was continuing to inquire whether Dr. Cutter could cosmetically do what I wanted and needed when Dr. Cutter took charge of my cosmetic destiny like a shark, which doesn't negotiate with its victim. It just comes up and proceeds to take the leg off of its victim without discussion. Dr. Donald Philbert's evaluation of Dr. Cutter's cosmetic work on me stated, "The miscommunication with the oral surgeon was sad."

The Medical Quality Assurance Commission needs to take immediate action against any nonrecognized medical doctor who has stated by his words and surgical actions that there are a lot of boards out there. The surgical doors have been left open to cause untold butchery on multitudes of unsuspecting cosmetic patients that the medical board have to be held accountable for. The medical board should not wait for more than one complaint in the same category against a medical doctor before they choose to wake up and immediately enact new laws prohibiting nonrecognized medical doctors from committing cosmetic crimes against unsuspecting patients.

I request that they terminate the current investigator unit chief, Arnold Richards, at the Medical Quality Assurance Commission, who denied opening a criminal investigation against Dr. Cutter, and hire a new one who will get aggressive regarding investigating any cry by victimized patients for a criminal investigation, as I repeatedly did without any action being taken. I was victimized, but I had difficulty coming up with the winning criminal combination of answers to satisfy the medical board and the investigator unit and its chief.

I know that the medical board failed to communicate what they were looking for from me to prove what Dr. Cutter had done to me, and I believe they should have called for a criminal investigation because I had requested one. To satisfy any suspicions and all possibilities of criminal actions taken toward the patient, the board should have the investigator unit meet with the medical doctor just to eliminate any criminal wrongdoing provided there is good evidence for an investigation. Besides being cosmetically violated and personally devastated, I dealt with ongoing confusion for years.

God says in His Word, "God is not the author of confusion but of peace" (1 Cor. 14:33).

I know that Dr. Cutter did a masterful job of assaulting my mind with mental blockages and blockades, most likely with a chemical to make certain that I had difficulties being able to solve the crimes committed against my person.

I know that Dr. Cutter found a way to desensitize my mind so that the doctor could help himself to my cosmetic and financial spoils without getting caught. Dr. Cutter was a cosmetic slacker and con artist, driven by power, greed, and control issues that motivated him to deceive, fool, and redirect the review board and investigator unit's attention away from the fact that he committed a highly calculated, sinister crime against me that would take me years to fully figure out.

I found that it took me between eight to nine years to fully understand exactly what Dr. Cutter had done to me. I know that Dr. Cutter was driven to devour my cosmetic and financial business like an anaconda when faced with an unsuspecting bunny rabbit. It attacks the rabbit to devour it whole without any hesitation. I wanted my cosmetic blueprint fulfilled, and Dr. Cutter wanted to add me to his medical statistics by fulfilling his cosmetic quota. It suddenly became the unskilled, unqualified, and nonspecialized cosmetic surgeon working on a multiple-surgery patient, who wanted and needed a Certified American Board Plastic Surgeon; the work ended in deplorable cosmetic results for me. After mentally desensitizing me, Dr. Cutter then forced me to solve the case of proving that I had truly been victimized by him.

Dr. Cutter had to know that he was putting me into an extremely difficult position of solving his cosmetic crimes against me so that the investigator unit and medical review board would take decisive action against him. Dr. Raymond Rockwell told me that he would consider it a crime if Dr. Cutter had left an orange peeling in my nose. I have come to the realization that the key thing the review board team and the investigator unit are looking for is if a medical doctor leaves behind an orange peeling, cosmetic knife, or screwdriver intentionally or by accident, and then they will determine it to be a crime.

That let me know that medical doctors are allowed to get away with various types of medical malpractice crimes provided the medical doctors do not leave behind any evidence to prove their crimes. If the patient isn't able to prove his criminal case to the medical board and to the investigator unit, he must find a medical doctor who is willing to go on record and say that the medical doctor didn't do what the patient wanted and needed. Most medical doctors are not willing to testify in court that another doctor committed a cosmetic crime against his patient—especially if the doctors live in the same state.

I have come to the realization that in Dr. Cutter's insatiable drive to deceive the medical board and the investigator unit, he became oblivious to my cosmetic interests. Dr. Cutter had to have concluded, "How can I go wrong with this cosmetic simpleton? He is a multiple-surgery patient. If I mess up, no one will notice."

Dr. Cutter was so hell-bent, determined, and strongly driven to dupe and deceive me into accepting that my raised and repositioned nose was normal, just like a shark suddenly causes its victim to unwillingly accept his missing leg and chewed-on body part. The victimized patient is suddenly forced to deal with the aftermath of all the mental, emotional, and irreparable cosmetic damages if the Certified American Board Plastic and Reconstruction surgeon is unsuccessful at repairing the physical characteristics by surgical revisions to his nose and ears.

Dr. Cutter told me twice, "I like you."

I didn't need any more counterfeit affection from Dr. Cutter as a means of deflecting serious questions from his victimized patient.

The more I experienced postsurgery professional and social rejections from my coworkers, passengers on my personnel carriers, churchgoers, and the general public, the more I became obsessive in my thoughts about Dr. Cutter.

It didn't matter what I found myself doing; I continuously reflected about Dr. Cutter and the sinister approach that Dr. Cutter had taken with me. I found myself talking to myself about Dr. Cutter at times, and I also found myself becoming angry about Dr. Cutter's slipshod approach, and methods of plundering my cosmetic and financial business. I knew unequivocally that I should not have to be dealing with all the painful and agonizing miseries on my life's plate just because one medical doctor wanted to deceive me, the medical board, and the investigator unit that his nonrecognized board status was just as qualified as are the medical specialists recognized on the twenty-four boards of ABMS.

I remained friendly toward my family, friends, and the passengers on the carrier routes I drove. After being mentally assaulted and cosmetically victimized, I found that the quality of my life had been significantly reduced because Dr. Cutter's actions against me were off the charts as to missing the mark when it came to meeting any standard of quality care and cosmetic procedures to match with the patient's expectations.

Simply put, Dr. Cutter's approach with me was cruel, criminal, and immoral.

I became continuously reflective regarding Dr. Cutter's slipshod cosmetic crime against me. I became obsessive about Dr. Cutter's approach with me, which was not something normal for a medical doctor to do. Even if Dr. Cutter's slam, bam, thank you, Kurtess Scone, for your cosmetic and financial business had turned out incredibly to be a beauty enhancement, it still would be a crime because of the inappropriate approach that Dr. Cutter had taken with me. Because of Dr. Cutter's aggressive approach toward me, I felt mentally and cosmetically violated. My person felt violated by Dr. Cutter because I was violated by him. No question about it.

I recall that my continuous reflective thoughts about Dr. Cutter twice brought an evil presence into my home. I realized that had I entered into and entertained the negative spirit to bring negative, harmful consequences to Dr. Cutter, I would have crossed the line of life to choose the opposite for Dr. Cutter.

I realized the evil presence that had been brought near was not thinking of me and Dr. Cutter's best interests. I rejected the evil spirit and his ultimate bidding and luring thoughts of harming Dr. Cutter.

God had to help me with my thought life. I have successfully been able to figure out exactly the things that Dr. Cutter did to me thanks to the Lord. I know what the medical board is looking for to prove what I experienced at the hands of Dr. Cutter. It has taken me quite a number of wasted years that I would never have had to painfully suffer had Dr. Cutter been willing to tell me the truth during our initial consultation. I went on a protracted spiritual fast, and I am convinced that the Lord revealed to me and or allowed me to see Dr. Cutter's actions in his dimly lit, presurgery room.

I saw Dr. Cutter turned sideways in a chair, and he began to rock back and forth with a big grin of triumph on his face while I was mentally impaired. I was able to witness Dr. Cutter move about his presurgery, mental-desensitization room and strategically place himself in different positions while I was only able to look on in mental silence. My recollections were like an old movie projector that would start and stop. I was frozen in my seat and totally unable to move when Dr. Cutter placed himself in his final presurgery position over to the right of where I was sitting. Dr. Cutter was intently staring at me as if to say, "I told you what I said I was going to do. Now what are you going to do?" I suddenly jumped up, trying to mentally grasp what Dr. Cutter was going to do to my nose. When I couldn't comprehend anything of Dr. Cutter's rhinoplasty plans for me, I closed my eyes in mental blankness and tension.

I eventually solved Dr. Cutter's crime against me with persistent mental evaluations; I continuously pressed forth to figure out the strange experience I had suffered and endured throughout the years. Dr. Cutter utilized mental blocks that prevented me from coming to an early and decisive criminal conclusion. I was able to solve the cosmetic bonanza puzzle concerning my nose, ears, and chin: Dr. Cutter waited until he moved me into an altered state of consciousness before he shared with me that he was going to raise and reposition my nose—two things that I absolutely didn't want, need, or expect cosmetically to be done to my nose to correct its definition. This scary, painful, and devastating move by Dr. Cutter against me, a totally unsuspecting client and patient, was clearly sinister and devious crimes in no uncertain terms. With God's help, I eventually solved Dr. Cutter's criminal cosmetic case that the medical board and investigator unit had willfully missed.

I was under Dr. Cutter's hypnosis and mind-control tactics. I would call this mental desensitization of Dr. Cutter's mental-control methods being in la-la land.

God allowed me to visually see black negative images, which had been imprinted on my memory bank when Dr. Cutter hit me with his psychological whammy. I didn't recall seeing these mental images when my mind first went blank after thinking about why Dr. Cutter hadn't told him up front of his plans to build up the bridge of my nose. I was given a vision by God of Dr. Cutter's presurgery actions in his presurgery, dimly lit room.

When I shared this information with the medical review board, it turned a blind eye and a deaf ear at taking any action against a cosmetic predator. It would require more time for me to know exactly what I had fully experienced at Dr. Cutter's surgical hands and what the medical board was looking for before they would take action against Dr. Cutter. Going on the factual basis of what I had experienced and was continuing to experience postsurgery, it felt like Dr. Cutter had shoved his cosmetic plans up into my subconscious mind, which I found was elusive to my analytical and inquisitive mind for years.

Scientists have discovered how to split the atom and to put a man on the moon. Had mankind been faithful to the will and plan of God Almighty, *He* would have made certain that we achieved far greater accomplishments than what mankind has been able to achieve down through the centuries. I am convinced that Dr. Cutter started to believe in his grandiose, narcissistic fantasy that he could tear down Dr. Lowell Piper's cosmetic work and Dr. Chris Kirtpatrick's plastic surgery work and rebuild my nose in an elevated position that was totally against my cosmetic blueprint for my nose.

Dr. Cutter rearranged and repositioned my nose, which became excruciatingly ugly to look at and painfully embarrassing and offensive to me and the general public to behold. Dr. Cutter would also tear down Dr. Christopher Smith's plastic surgery work on my ears and chin, again positively against my cosmetic blueprint and interests for my ears. The chin fell into Dr. Cutter's specialty, and I admit that after I shaved my beard off about a year later, my chin looked pretty good. But for my nose and ears, as I reiterated, Dr. Cutter was not a precision-skilled specialist as a plastic surgeon would be. Dr. Cutter's postsurgery results became a horrifying nightmare for me to painfully experience, endure, and suffer.

I recall that my wife, Lorena, and I began watching *A Haunting* programs on television together. As a married couple, we found that although we were Christians in our faith in Christ Jesus and I knew that we shouldn't be watching reenactments of actual true events that have taken place in homes around the world, we were curious to watch these programs and see what the unsuspecting people experienced. These spooky programs portray the works of demonic activities that have occurred in peoples' homes and lives. Lorena and I got into watching these programs on a frequent basis until I had a spiritual dream that had a demonic manifestation of a person laughing at me in a mocking manner.

I shared my dream with my sister Marlie and how I remembered seeing Dr. Cutter doing this same type of mocking me, with a sinister grin on his face as if he had conquered me, in a spiritual vision from the Lord. I asked the Lord to help me know what Dr. Cutter had done to me. Marlie told me that the devil was using this program to come against me, just as Dr. Cutter had on the day of my surgeries. Marlie told me that I needed to stop watching these programs, and thank God, Lorena and I closed the door on the devil's work by putting an end to watching the scary programs together.

I reflected back on the words that I remember Dr. Cutter said to me as I followed the medical doctor from one consultation room into an adjacent, separate room approximately three months postsurgery. I had come back in with my coworker Denise to have a talk with the doctor about the adverse changes he had made to my facial features.

Dr. Cutter asked me, "Didn't I tell you that I was going to raise and reposition your nose?"

I boldly responded to Dr. Cutter, "No, you didn't."

I remember that suddenly Dr. Cutter had a surprised look on his face when his patient spoke to the doctor in such a forceful manner in responding to his question. I now understand the first half of Dr. Cutter's crime had taken place inside of this very room, which turned out to be his presurgery, dimly lit, psycho deception tactics, hypnotic whammy room, where he assaulted my brain before my surgeries. I now realize that postsurgery Dr. Cutter wanted me to have a hypnotic flashback, wherein I would be able to recall the doctor's presurgery words spoken to me. Dr. Cutter found that utilizing suggestive words and actions did not work on me.

I have come to the realization that when Dr. Cutter conducted his psycho deception tactics of hypnosis on me, he was in league with spiritual darkness that was willing to hurt me in a negative impacting and destructive way. Dr. Cutter was not going to play fair with me, just like the devil is not willing to play fair with his victims.

Satan rules in spiritual darkness; the Bible says he is the god of this world and the prince of the power of the air. He is the spirit that now works in the sons of disobedience, says the apostle Paul in Ephesians chapter two. I have come to the realization that Dr. Cutter didn't act alone; whether he knew it or not at the time of his cosmetic scam operation, he became a tool of the devil to seek, steal, and if possible destroy my life, which had been dedicated to the Lord by my father, Benjamin, and my mother, Jessica.

God wanted to be the only one who brought true satisfaction into my life and character by having me look to Him to make something beautiful in my life. God wanted to do a good work in me, and He didn't want me to be hurt by the selfish actions of a cosmetic surgeon. It was not God's will that I was victimized by an unqualified cosmetic surgeon; rather, it was God's will to keep me from harm.

I have come to the realization that Dr. Cutter, like so many other criminals, has been able to escape man's justice on earth, but if he doesn't repent of the error of his ways, he won't be able to escape heaven's justice in the future. There is a day of reckoning coming, which the Bible speaks of, wherein each person will give account of himself to God for the life that he or she has lived.

Mankind may not like to think about the fact that we are all accountable to a powerful, all-knowing God and we are responsible for our actions toward our fellow man, whether we like to think of it or not.

God says in His Word that "He is not willing that any should perish, but that all should come to repentance" (2 Pet. 3:9).

Dr. Cutter's actions against me in the nineties have not been ignored and overlooked by our loving God, who is the ultimate judge of the people of this world.

I do not wish Dr. Cutter God's wrath and judgment in the future. I would like to see Dr. Cutter repent of his sinister actions and become a God-fearing man who treats his fellow man with respect, dignity, and honor. I have come to recognize that Dr. Cutter applied the iron will of his cosmetic agenda to me, and I would like to see the iron will of justice applied to Dr. Cutter for his criminal wrongdoings. May the iron will of justice prevail in my case against Dr. Cutter.

My coworker Denise encouraged me to write down notes that came to my mind regarding Dr. Cutter. I accepted Denise's advice and began writing down copious notes of what I could remember happening to me pre- and postsurgery. I knew that Dr. Cutter's approach toward myself was not morally ethical, but it was even something more devious in nature, which would take me years to totally figure out exactly what I had experienced that the medical board and the investigator unit were looking for. I know now what they are requiring from each victimized patient, but I know that when the medical and dental boards even hear that a medical doctor isn't a recognized cosmetic surgeon with the right certification and credentials, they should immediately call for a criminal investigation against that doctor. If the patient says or sends in a complaint that he or she was violated by a medical doctor, the medical board should instantly check to see if the doctor is certified by the American Board of Plastic Surgery and find out if the cosmetic surgeon isn't on a recognized board. If the medical doctor isn't on any one of the twenty-four boards of medical specialties defined by the ABMS, they should begin an immediate criminal investigation against the surgeon because they will then have full knowledge that something of a sinister nature has happened to that unsuspecting patient.

I have come to the realization that there are certain medical doctors who are willing to desensitize and mentally stun the minds of patients in order to get a quick confession from an unsuspecting patient. This is exactly what I experienced at the hands of Dr. Cutter, who tried to deceive the medical board and the investigator unit from taking any action against him. After I was duped, deceived, conned, and scammed, Dr. Cutter pulled himself back in line with the ethics board's policies as a caring physician, while the patient was left in a sea of mental confusion as to what happened to me. When I made my formal complaint to the medical board, I must have been perceived as negative, possibly a hypochondriac, and/or a crazy lunatic. The medical doctor carries on his professional practice as if he had not committed a heinous crime against me.

When the medical board reviewed my complaint letters, Dr. Cutter evaluated his patient as having psychological issues, and the medical board bought into his psychological evaluation of my mental health, although he was not a qualified psychologist nor a psychiatrist, and simply closed the case. Dr. Cutter went so far as to recommend counseling for me to cover his criminal actions and to deceive the investigator unit and medical board into thinking that he is a caring physician. I know better by Dr. Cutter's actions toward me; I know that Dr. Cutter recommended counseling for me only when I began to question what had happened to me cosmetically. I came to recognize that Dr. Cutter's actions were reactionary to my questions in an effort to cover his crimes, and not proactive as a caring physician postsurgery toward me personally.

I found that there were certain things that I would do postsurgery that momentarily helped me to forget about my cosmetic victimization by Dr. Cutter. I worked on isolating myself from many social settings for years, and I wrote many complaint letters to the medical board regarding Dr. Cutter's approach toward me. I found that talking with friends helped me to forget about the pain of my disfigurement and horrible victimization by a cosmetic surgeon who never should have touched my nose and ears. I didn't tell my family for years what had happened to me because it was too painfully embarrassing and humiliating to be talking about such sensitive personal issues.

I also found that it helped me to listen to Christian, bluegrass, and country music to take my mind off my suffering. I would also play my banjo for long periods of time to help me concentrate on something other than my mental, emotional, and cosmetic ordeal. I remember reading in Katharine A. Phillips's book *The Broken Mirror* about individuals who have serious preoccupations and have obsessive thoughts over the slightest physical flaw, which most people simply overlook. There are a lot of people who become reclusive from social interaction and purposefully avoid making wholesome relationships because of their obsessive preoccupation with their physical imperfections and their looks in general. I came to realize that there are a lot of hurting people who suffer on a daily basis because they have great difficulties with their physical appearance. I also recognize that many people suffer unnecessarily because of what unqualified medical doctors have done to them cosmetically. These medical doctors want to improve on their limited training skills so they end up using the patient to practice on with their nonrecognized training and end up making some extra money at the same time. The patient then is left to suffer unnecessarily, possibly for years.

I purposely remained on certain carrier routes for William County Carrier Company because I knew the passengers were familiar with my postsurgery physical appearance. I knew that if I were to pick new routes, the passengers would have to get over the initial shock of seeing me for the first time on each of the routes I chose.

I have experienced a negative life-impacting inferiority complex, which has been abusive in nature to my personal, social, neighborhood, and professional relationships. I would like to thank all the passengers, customers, and clients, and general public who have accepted me with my physical characteristics just the way they are. I would like to offer my humble and sincere apology to all my professional coworkers, the passengers, and the general public for any disconcerting, disfigured cosmetic physical feature appearances that have caused a great number of people to recoil or simply look away because they were mentally and emotionally uncomfortable and embarrassed when looking at me.

I know for a 100 percent fact that I have been misunderstood by different groups of people over the years. They have misunderstood my friendliness and my smile, which are a positive reflection of the life of Jesus Christ in my heart and life. My friendliness and smile are an outward sign, expression, and manifestation of the inward work of the Spirit of Christ. I have also used my smile to compensate for the cosmetic changes that have been painfully difficult to live and work with, to say the least. By the responses and actions I have gotten from plenty of men and women who strangely disappear from riding my carrier routes after they have ridden my personnel carrier one or more times, I have concluded that they either abhor my physical appearance, fell victim to the rumor mill or gossip stories about me, or erroneously thought that I flirted with them or someone they have heard about. The actual fact and truth of the matter is that I enjoy being friendly and talking with men and women of all ages if they are open to a short or lengthy conversation. Certain individuals act like they are anticommunication, and they come onto my carrier and exit my carrier coach without saying a word of thanks for my driving service. I am definitely not flirting with men or women when I talk to individual passengers on my carrier routes. I recognize that many carrier drivers choose to keep a low profile and not get into communicating with the passengers to avoid being distracted, resulting in having a preventable accident.

I have experienced that many of my coworkers employed with William County Carrier Company avoid making eye contact with me. I have had fellow employees give me a look over when I have signed in for work throughout the years. I have had different people over the years wonder what my ethnic background is. My supervisor at Rolland Carrier site wondered if I was Italian. I was caught off guard because of the unusual question when signing in for work, but I found myself telling my superior in jest that I had a Roman nose.

Lukas, my supervisor, said, "Roman is Italian."

I didn't try to correct Lukas Palmer on my Norwegian ethnicity on my father's side and Scottish and Irish on my mother's side of the family. I realize that many people seem to be puzzled by my physical appearance by the things they have communicated to me over the years. I know that I am a real work of art, with other medical doctors taking my nose in one direction and Dr. Cutter taking my nose in an elevated position and then rearranging it completely opposite of what I wanted, needed, and expected cosmetically.

I went to see an attorney who worked for an established law firm in Union. The attorney asked a woman who worked at the law firm what she thought of my postsurgery nose job and whether she could see any problems with it. The woman became evasive about whether she could observe any problems with my nose. I picked up on the fact that the female employee, when called upon by the attorney, couldn't respond truthfully if she said, "It's a good-looking nose. I don't see anything wrong with it. He should be very pleased with the cosmetic surgeon's work." I found that I didn't care for the attorney's approach of seeking for a negative response regarding my nose from the employee without asking me whether I was open for the woman's evaluation cold turkey.

When I called up the same attorney at a later time to inform him that I believed Dr. Cutter had utilized hypnosis on me, the attorney wanted me to tell him how Dr. Cutter had done that. I discovered that I couldn't define or describe exactly how Dr. Cutter had gone about hypnotizing me at the time. I recall that the attorney came across to me as rather cold, psychologically pushy, and pressing me for answers that I hadn't been able to completely figure out at that point. I never called the attorney back after that.

Judging by my experiences, I am sure that Dr. Cutter knows that most victims will mentally give up the struggle to pursue justice to its final conclusion. Dr. Cutter knows that a victimized patient has to persevere through the maze of mental confusion to mentally persuade the medical review board and the investigator unit to sit up and take notice of criminal acts of true victimization.

I had a good talk with my friend Leroy O'Hara concerning Dr. Cutter's motivations for committing cosmetic crimes against me. Leroy expressed to me that the doctor would have to be crazy to do so. I initially responded in the affirmative by saying, "He was crazy." I am persuaded that Dr. Cutter was cunning in his actions toward me on the day of surgery since he knew that he wasn't specialized in the nose and ears, and yet he forged ahead to perform cosmetic surgeries on my physical characteristics regardless of the consequences and my cosmetic interests. No patient wants a nonrecognized medical doctor surgically doing the complete opposite of what he or she cosmetically wants and needs.

I remember talking to a woman who worked for the Medical Quality Assurance Commission a number of years ago. I don't even know her name, but I remember telling her that I felt like I was cosmetically raped by Dr. Cutter. I related that although I wasn't a woman, I know what it feels like to be raped. I experienced a mental, cosmetic, emotional, and financial violation to my whole person by Dr. Cutter, but I wasn't able to explain or describe everything to the woman at the time. The woman was silent at first as she listened on the phone to my horrible experience. She soon wanted to get off the phone after she heard my negative description of what I had experienced in real life by Dr. Cutter.

My friend Leroy couldn't understand why I would allow this event with Dr. Cutter to trouble me for the last seven years. I know that my friend never experienced what I have been suffering and dealing with psychologically, spiritually, emotionally, and in my social and personal relationships. I don't fault the woman at the MQAC nor my friend for not understanding the terrible cosmetic and financial ordeal that I have experienced and suffered needlessly because of a greedy and uncaring cosmetic surgeon.

I have come to realize over a number of wasted years that my experience with Dr. Cutter is because I was deceived, duped, scammed, and conned by Dr. Cutter cosmetically and financially. I only wish I could have seen what the medical review board and the investigator unit were looking for a lot sooner. I recognize that I was so painfully devastated mentally and cosmetically, besides being in mental confusion for years, that I had great difficulty trying to pinpoint exactly what the medical board was looking for. Personally I believe that I made a number of good points that should have moved the medical board and the investigator unit to call for a criminal investigation because I requested one to take place. They needed me to emphatically say that I didn't have a partial or a full understanding of what Dr. Cutter was going to do to me cosmetically presurgery. The previous statement is 100 percent factually true.

I would like to know how many patients are allowed to die under the care of a physician before someone takes action. Dr. Cutter had patient complaint number five under his dental board die on him. I discovered that Dr. Cutter had another patient whose treatment ended in death or in injury. When I inquired if the disclosure representative could provide that information to me, he let me know that he couldn't do that. It is pretty scary to be dealing with a doctor who has any patient die under his or her care, finding out this information, as I had done, only postsurgery.

I am convinced that Dr. Cutter and other nonrecognized medical doctors are accidents, medical malpractice cases, lawsuits, injuries, and even deaths just waiting to happen because they hold the power of life and death over their patients. Whether they know how to control that power or not depends on a number of factors. A big factor is whether they have a qualified anesthesiologist or whether they are conserving on money by not hiring a qualified anesthesiologist. I encourage the reader to ask a lot of questions of the medical doctor that you plan on having cosmetic surgery with and to talk to a number of patients who have had cosmetic surgery on the same body part that you want surgery on for yourself.

I was informed by the Medical Quality Assurance Commission that they can't judge on the basis of cosmetic results. I urge the medical commissions, societies, and medical review teams throughout the land to change their rulings, upheld by the medical boards, to include cosmetic results as evidence for a criminal investigation. Where there is smoke, there is fire. If a nonrecognized medical doctor elects to forge ahead and cosmetically do things that one or more medical doctors recognizes as a misunderstanding, misinterpretation, miscommunication, not what the patient wanted or needed, and so on, then the medical review teams and the investigator unit need to call for an immediate criminal investigation regarding the nonspecialized medical doctor—especially if the patient is experiencing postsurgery symptoms of short-term or long-term confusion, difficulties in retrieving memories, and difficulties when thinking about what has transpired with a medical doctor.

On the day of my surgeries, I was not experiencing mental confusion. Postsurgery I experienced the above symptoms, along with mental tension for years, as a result of my encounter with Dr. Cutter. Postsurgery I remember telling a friend that my brain had been freeze-dried in blackness. I know for a 100 percent fact that these symptoms are not normal, and the Medical Quality Assurance Commission and the William County Medical Society need to recognize that there are predators in the medical field who are out to deceive the medical review teams and every investigator unit put on each individual case.

I have come to the realization that the social and professional rejections I have suffered throughout the years are powerful evidence that cosmetic and financial crimes were committed against me by Dr. Cutter. I have come to the realization that juries are not sympathetic toward multiple-surgery patients in the state of Washington, and neither is the general public sympathetic regarding cosmetic victims who suffer in silence when observed and witnessed carrying on their business or dealing with matters as successfully as they can under their victimized circumstances.

I discovered that the general public in Union and the area surrounding the city in many cases have had a negative reaction to my physical appearance. I know that this has not been due to merely psychological issues on my part. I have done my own testing of my victimized situation by acting cool, calm, and collected out in public places versus times where I had had more of a psychological stigma in which I had had some major personal issues due to which I would rather not be around others, feeling uncomfortable when out with the general public because of being rejected or stared at in public. Being out in social settings has not been a pleasant experience for me to publicly deal with throughout the years. In most cases, I have preferred to remain at home and not go out in full view of the general public since my surgeries with Dr. Cutter and subsequent postsurgery revisions with Dr. Rockwell.

Each time I underwent a cosmetic revision by Dr. Raymond Rockwell, I had to go through the postrevision changes to my physical appearance. I had to endure the postsurgery swelling and any new physical facial changes that the general public hadn't seen before.

I began to think that the general public, which had observed what I looked like before any revision work, must have grown weary of each subtle or major variation that became noticeably objectionable to my physical looks. It became especially difficult if I observed that the revision change or changes to my physical facial characteristic was not going to enhance my new look nor appear to look normal in appearance. It positively didn't help matters if I noticed that people were not comfortable with the physical changes I now possessed.

I have purposefully put my hand up directly under my nose while driving my personal vehicle by myself to prevent people from noticing my unpleasant physical appearance. I have also many times driven my private automobile holding a plastic or paper cup to cover my nose from being noticed by the general public. Someone reading this might think that I shouldn't even care what people think about my physical appearance no matter how physically objectionable I may look. For the reader, the above sounds like an easy answer that they might observe if they were cosmetically victimized, but I do care what people think and how they react to my physical looks.

I discovered that Dr. Rockwell wanted $17,700.00 for the initial set of revisions done to my physical characteristics. My initial $120.00 consultation fee was included into the total cost for the corrective revisions. With having to pay for my airfare, rental car, and motel costs, it has run into some big bucks for me to undergo each set of revision surgeries over the years since my encounter with Dr. Cutter.

I have had to deal with the embarrassment, shame, and humiliation from the changes I have gone through with every new change to my face. This has added to the difficulty for me to be seen and observed by the general public under various circumstances and by the passengers who ride my carrier routes. I know that I have not been careless in my actions to offend, embarrass, and hurt any passenger regardless of his or her skin color because I have made an attempt to be kind, considerate, and polite with all of my passengers.

I would like for the good people of every ethnic group to know that my actions and nonactions when it comes to my mannerisms on my personnel carrier routes have been seriously negatively impacted by what I have suffered psychologically, emotionally, and cosmetically at the hands of Dr. Cutter. I sincerely and honestly would like to apologize to anyone and everyone who have been offended by my uncharacteristic mannerisms and actions on all of my carrier routes.

I recognize that I have depended and relied on my good friend Richard Dandy to help me with personal business and shopping. I have suffered with inferiority and self-image issues, besides having a psychological stigma that has characterized my personal life as not being normal to the general public.

I know that my victimization by Dr. Cutter was not an accident, but a cunningly planned cosmetic and financial crime by a sinister medical doctor. I wasn't supposed to wake up to my troubling cosmetic ordeal; I know now by what I have experienced that should I not have awakened to Dr. Cutter's deranged actions against me, I would continue having mental illness, in which one goes back and forth between periods of mania and periods of depression. I was supposed to have manic-depressive psychological issues, wherein I wasn't intended to mentally wake up to Dr. Cutter's mentally sick cosmetic scheme and scam committed against me.

I was meant to remain in the dark concerning the cruel, criminal, and immoral crimes forced on me by a psychotic sociopath. This way Dr. Cutter would slink back into his normal role as a caring cosmetic physician who didn't do one thing wrong during his professional practice against his victimized patient. I know better, but the medical board and the investigator unit have refused to recognize the evidence of the criminal elements in my case. I have heard that he has a dental practice in the city he currently resides in. I was informed that he has been on probation for four years. I wasn't informed of the reason behind his probation. Perhaps this could be the year that I and others will finally receive news that justice will be appropriately served by the medical board and the investigator unit rendering disciplinary or termination action against Dr. Cutter. I know that justice has not prevailed up until now in my case.

I recognize from a Christian perspective that Dr. Cutter was used by the devil on the day of my surgeries as a tool to assault my spiritual man and my physical body. I recognize that my real enemy is the devil, according to Jesus Christ, the greatest historian and authority on spiritual matters and on earthly matters. (See John 8:44.)

The Bible records in Ephesians 6:12, "For we do not wrestle against flesh and blood, but against principalities, and powers, against the rulers of the darkness of this age, against spiritual hosts of wickedness in the heavenly places." I have come to realize that Dr. Cutter was used by the devil as a vessel to try to destroy my life with abusive cosmetic surgeries that Dr. Cutter knew he didn't have the specialty for. I know that the devil is the real culprit and scoundrel who committed the cosmetic and financial crimes against me through Dr. Cutter. I have come to recognize that Dr. Cutter, who was not specialized in the nose and ears, was willing and perfectly ready to do some more cutting on me because he believed he could get away with it. I would like to see the iron will of justice applied to Dr. Cutter's actions and lack of subspecialty training in the nose and ears, which he applied cunningly against my physical characteristics.

I recall how Dr. Cutter was adroit at keeping me mentally questioning and starved for more detailed and specific information presurgery as to exactly what he was going to do to my physical characteristics. I was left feeling confused, abused, and victimized when I continuously reflected on the words and actions of Dr. Cutter postsurgery. I know that Dr. Cutter felt pretty assured of himself when committing his crimes against me. I know that Dr. Cutter didn't expect me to have a good memory regarding his actions against me. I know that Dr. Cutter was going for a quick confession from me, and then he could simply move on as a caring physician of cosmetic surgery for first-time patients only. He would also continue to specialize in dentistry, and no one would be the wiser, including the medical board and the investigator unit in regard to his cosmetic and financial crimes committed against me and others.

I see Dr. Cutter as a dangerous spectator at the 2008 Summer Olympic games in Beijing, China, who would intentionally trip an Olympic runner out of spite because he thought he could get away with it. He would then pull his leg back quickly without being witnessed by other people attending the games, while the injured athlete would lose out on his quest for Olympic gold.

I threw a monkey wrench into the operational gears of Dr. Cutter's cosmetic surgery machinery when I sent in my complaints against him. I came to the painful realization that Dr. Cutter's cosmetic approach was unethical and that he needed to be investigated for committing cosmetic crimes against me. The investigation never took place, but I felt that I needed to warn the medical board about Dr. Cutter's cruel professional practice and scary cosmetic results that patients would be seriously hurt from. Dr. Cutter acted post-surgery like he couldn't believe I was able to have any recall about his actions toward me. He also seemed to be pretty assured of himself postsurgery, as if he was pleased that he had had the opportunity to cosmetically work on me. I have come to recognize and realize that Dr. Cutter should have never been given that opportunity in the first place.

I know that there is a crisis in Victimized, USA, concerning medical malpractice cases, wherein medical doctors who are not skilled and qualified to surgically perform specialized plastic surgery procedures on patients who need careful reconstructive cosmetic work are still allowed to operate. The medical board has allowed these unqualified medical doctors to make some extra money by cosmetically working on multiple-surgery patients who do not want, need, or expect first-time cosmetic work repeated over again in an elevated position. I know that the time for the medical board to change their policies to prevent and restrict cosmetic surgeons who have a nonrecognized status from hurting unsuspecting patients is long overdue.

My friend Tommy Ray recognizes that the surefire way that the medical board could eliminate the medical malpractice problem is to have all medical doctors videotape their consultations. This way every trusting patient would be guaranteed and ensured the medical doctor he or she is dealing with will treat the patient with the most respect, dignity, and utmost care. By videotaping the consultations, the medical doctors will have to be on their best behavior at all times and not be allowed to get away with outright medical malpractice.

The videotapes would be done with DVD discs, and the patient would be given a copy for review prior to the patient's scheduled date of surgery. The medical doctor who might want to alter the videotape to his advantage would be prevented from doing so when the medical doctor, patient, and the patient's family, attorney, or adult guardian all have the opportunity to review the exchange between the doctor and his or her trusting patient on the video.

The medical board, review teams, and investigator unit would be sent a copy of the agreed-upon type of surgery or surgeries before the medical doctor would be permitted to proceed with the patient's surgery or surgeries. Had the above policy been adopted by the medical board and the legislators in the state of Washington, I would not have been victimized by Dr. Cutter.

I have enjoyed over the years the many attractions that Union has to offer. I have enjoyed Christian events, sporting events, concerts, musical events, parks, and parades. I have appreciated watching the Blue Angels perform their amazing flight patterns and routines when they have been in the greater Union area. I have enjoyed the wonderful creations of God and man throughout my many years. The one situation that I haven't appreciated dealing with is the negative repercussions I have experienced from the general public; I know they do not understand what I have been dealing with as a man on my mental, emotional, and relationship plate. I have come to the realization that the social and professional repercussions have not been a total consequence of my own actions.

I have also come to realize that I am partly to blame for my social rejections because I have been far too open, free, and trusting of people in a negative environment, where to be socially indifferent and apathetic is acceptable in society. I also recognize that I have had conversations about my personal life with the general public on my personnel carriers, whereas many carrier drivers want to maintain a private, anonymous relationship with their passengers. I have become known by name by many of my carrier passengers as a caring, compassionate, considerate, and kindhearted carrier driver. I appreciate the people who have made me feel accepted just the way I am, the way I look, and the way I act as a man in a negative world.

After my surgeries with Dr. Cutter, I recall how my passengers on my carrier routes reacted negatively toward me. When I would look in the direction of my exiting customers wanting off my carrier shuttle, I observed how the passengers would repulsedly look at me and quickly want to exit my coach without saying a word of "thanks, driver."

From a worldly perspective, I recognize that the world loves its own and seeks to glorify, approve, and worship physical beauty. From a Christian perspective, I recognize that my fight is not with the passengers who do not approve of my physical appearance, but my warfare is with the principalities of darkness influencing clients to think and react negatively toward me. I recognize that the customers' negative reactions toward me should not be taken personally.

I contacted KOMO 4 news station in Seattle to talk with Joey Cunningham concerning my victimization story. Joey told me that he was willing to air my story provided the Medical Quality Assurance Commission had found that the medical doctor was in the wrong. Once again, I found myself stuck in my victimization from telling my story, and I was not able to tell my account of true events wherein I was used and abused by a medical doctor.

I knew I was blocked from moving on with my life because the Medical Quality Assurance Commission had not even requested Dr. Cutter to respond to my complaint against him. I felt that I needed closure to my victimization verdict prompted by Dr. Cutter's own actions, and the medical review board and the investigator unit closed and kept closed my case against Dr. Cutter, even after repeated requests for a reconsideration and a rehearing to reopen my case. To my knowledge, the medical board had granted me a reconsideration to open my case against Dr. Cutter, only to have it closed after a period of time. I know I am a victim of a cosmetic predator and my case warrants having a reconsideration based on all the evidence I have provided to the medical review board. Perhaps my book will bring some attention to my sad case, and I will soon find myself closer to the end of my long ordeal as a cosmetic victim.

I know that actual crimes were committed against me by Dr. Cutter, but the Medical Quality Assurance Commission, representing the state, didn't see it that way, nor did they believe his actions were a crime committed against me. Obviously their investigation was not very thorough. I dare to differ totally from the commission's investigator unit's ruling and stand up for what I firmly know, am convinced of, and am persuaded of for a 100 percent fact that definite crimes were committed against my personhood by Dr. Cutter's intentional criminal acts of medical malpractice. Instead of simply feeling that crimes were committed against me by Dr. Cutter, I *know* that crimes were committed against me, no matter whether the state, commission, law, police, or the highest courts in the land of Victimized, USA, stated otherwise. I am a survivor of medical malpractice crimes committed against me by Dr. Cutter, and I dare to challenge anyone to prove otherwise. Those of you reading this are probably aware of others who have suffered from medical malpractice.

I contacted a number of libraries regarding medical malpractice from a patient's perspective. I was informed that there wasn't a single book from a patient's perspective. I decided to contact an attorney's office out of the yellow pages to see if they knew of a book that was written from a patient's perspective. The paralegal who answered the phone didn't know of any such book, so she placed me on hold to ask her attorney if he might know of any medical malpractice book from a patient's perspective. When the paralegal came back on the line, she informed me that there wasn't any such book that the attorney knew of. I was informed that there are plenty of books written on medical malpractice that doctors and attorneys refer to concerning different case procedures, but none are written specifically from a patient's perspective. I decided that it was high time that a good book needed to be written from a patient's perspective on medical malpractice because of all the innocent people who are being hurt, used, abused, exploited, and victimized by medical doctors who are taking advantage of naïve, unsuspecting patients.

There are unsuspecting consumers who lack the knowledge of what they might expect in regard to postsurgery cosmetic results from nonrecognized, unqualified surgeons; they want the same cosmetic results as one would get from Certified American Board of Plastic Surgery medical doctors. The nonrecognized medical surgeons certified by the ABMS and the ABPS want financial compensation as their more skilled colleagues do. It wasn't my field of endeavor and expertise to know all of Dr. Cutter's fields of specialized training when I first saw his full-page ad. If I call 911, I safely assume and expect to find qualified, trained personnel who are competent in their field, whether they be ambulance, police, or fire department personnel, without having to check into their credentials. When they show up responding to the emergency call, I don't stop them and make them tell me all of their training before they proceed. It is only reasonable to expect the professional personnel who respond to my emergency call are well qualified to handle the serious circumstance they happen to encounter. The unskilled medical surgeons can only hope for the best, or they have to become masters of their own cosmetic world and simply tell their cosmetic subjects that they are going to like it. Whether he or she does like the postsurgery cosmetic results or not is up to the individual patient.

I painfully discovered that Dr. Cutter's cosmetic results were horrid and horrible for myself and the general public to look at. I hope to save the reader the same unpleasant fate as prescribed and dictated by the cosmetic surgeon who disfigured my nose and ears. The painful cosmetic results were realized gradually postsurgery for me, and then repeated over and over in my mind day in and day out for years. With each corrective surgery revision by Dr. Raymond Rockwell, a plastic surgeon who I came to realize is a genuine expert on the subject of cosmetic and reconstruction surgeries, I was again and again reminded that Dr. Cutter was not the skilled cosmetic surgeon I was searching for in the nineties, but he still ended up performing triple play surgeries on my nose, ears, and chin. The painful postsurgery results were for me scary to say the least.

I saw Pastor Alvarez on Trinity Broadcasting Network one day, and I heard about the creative miracles that were taking place in his church in Miami, Florida. I decided to fly down to Miami to get in on the wonderful things God was doing by His Holy Spirit in real people's lives during these current times. I put in for my vacation pick at work in the spring. I initially flew to Chicago, Illinois, and then I caught my second flight to Miami. I signed the papers for a rental car at the Miami Airport, and I drove around Miami for a while before driving down to the Rodeway Inn Motel in Homestead, Florida, where I had made reservations.

I found that it was a good experience for me to attend the large Apostolic Faith Center on a number of occasions during my time spent in Miami, Florida, and I was able to have Pastor Juan Alvarez actually pray for me outside of the large edifice on the church property. I appreciated having Pastor Alvarez listen attentively to my request for my nose to come down, and the man of God prayed a straightforward prayer that my nose would come down. He called for it to happen as he spoke forth prophetically in the presence of witnesses.

I didn't see my nose come down as a small mountain moving from one elevated position to another lower position as I was hoping would happen while I stood in front of Pastor Alvarez. God would use Dr. Raymond Rockwell to fulfill the prayer of the man of God during a surgical procedure in Los Angeles, California, in a partial way. Since Dr. Rockwell is not the God of supernatural restoration, he could only fulfill my creative miracle expectation in a partial sense through a series of corrective rhinoplasty revision procedures. I thank God for the reconstruction surgeries from which I benefited. I recognize that God uses creative miracles to accomplish His will on earth and He also uses the surgical skills of reconstruction plastic surgeons to bring about healing and wholeness into the realm of human suffering.

While visiting Florida, I took time to drive through the Florida Everglades National Park in my rental car, and I also drove down to Key

West on a separate beautiful spring day. I took in the state's amazing scenery traveling on Highway 1 south of Florida City. I enjoyed the beautiful Atlantic Ocean blue waters, and I drove across the seven-mile bridge stretched above the vast ocean blue-green waters. I kept driving south until I eventually reached the quaint city of Key West, with all of its attractive shops and businesses for every visiting tourist to enjoy browsing through. I was very much conscious of my appearance, and I decided to remain in my vehicle while taking in as many of the pleasant sights that Key West had to offer before heading back north to the Rodeway Inn Motel in Homestead, Florida.

On my final day in Homestead, I checked out of the motel and started to drive north to connect with Highway I-75. I continued driving through the state of Florida on I-75 all the way to Atlanta, Georgia. I had a semitruck barreling along right behind me on a dark Georgian night. I wasn't going to allow the truck driver intimidate me into driving at an excessive rate of speed above and beyond the posted speed limit. I knew the truck driver didn't know that I was a professional carrier driver, who wasn't going to become overly nervous as Dennis Weaver had in the movie *Duel* because of the truck driver's intimidating actions.

Eventually I made a pit stop in a rest area for a restroom break. Once I was back on the road again, I stopped for gas in Atlanta, where I was able to acquire driving directions from a helpful African American woman to Pastor Creflo Dollar's church in College Park, which is twenty minutes from Atlanta. I have appreciated listening to Pastor Dollar on Trinity Broadcasting Network. I discovered the church was closed that night, but I had a security guard invite me in to the large, impressive administration building of Dollar's ministry. The guard was very kindhearted to me and gave me a couple of ministry audiocassette tapes to listen to. I appreciated the security guard's cordial personality representing World Changers Church and the kind invitation to stay in Atlanta for a few days so I could take in an inspirational church service. I decided to continue my drive north and not hold up for a few days in Atlanta to enjoy the large city and to experience Pastor Dollar's teaching at one of their church services. Before leaving College Park and Atlanta, I was able to drive around the large megachurch estate area and catch a look at Dollar's 8,400-seat congregational church in the dark of night before I headed back to I-75 north.

Once I was back on I-75, I kept driving north until I decided to get some sleep in a rest area outside of Chattanooga, Tennessee. Upon waking up to a warm, sunny day, I continued my scenic drive up to Nashville, Tennessee. I drove around Nashville for some time, experiencing the city's sights such as Music Row and other interesting landmarks known to Nashville folk. I had driven around Nashville for quite some time, but I never was able to find the Grand Old Opry or Opryland, USA, as I hoped to. I needed to have someone with the Country Music Hall of Fame show me exactly where I needed to go in order to see the famous country music entertainment hall that has been the center of scores and scores of talented musicians and entertainers.

As I drove out of Nashville, Tennessee, on Highway 24, I observed the massive traffic congestion heading back into Nashville and beyond. When I saw the extended lineup of semitrucks in traffic, I was grateful I was leaving town rather than trying to work my way into the big city during rush hour. I continued driving to Paducah, Kentucky. I then worked my way eastward over to Highway 60 to Springfield, Missouri, where I held up for the night in a motel.

I was doing my very best to take in all the scenic sights of this great country that I could during my trip back home to the Pacific Northwest. I would look to my right and then to my left, not wanting to miss out on any of my traveling scenic adventures. I drove around Springfield for a long time trying to locate the Springfield Assembly of God Headquarters; my parents had paid tithes to the Christian organization throughout the years. Unfortunately I never did find the Assembly of God Headquarters with all of my driving around the beautiful city. While I drove around Springfield, I could understand why so many people wanted to live there, because it appeared to be a lovely city. As I was heading out of town, I observed the large James River Assembly of God Church with its rather impressive edifice.

I headed south on Highway 65 to Branson, Missouri, where I drove around the city looking at all the entertainment centers where live shows were held at different times throughout the day. I never took in any of the entertainment shows, which I could have, and I didn't even go into the Roy Rogers Museum, with Roy's horse, Trigger, rearing up high in the air out in front of the museum. My mother, Jessica Scone, always hoped that all of our family could go to Branson together someday to enjoy a great time of good entertainment. Unfortunately Benjamin Scone passed away at ninety-four years of age. Benjamin is now in heaven with Jesus, whom he preached about and wanted men, women, boys, and girls to meet and know Him. Benjamin is now forever in the presence of God, the Holy Angels, and all the saints above. He will be missed by his family, who loved and appreciated him.

When I left Branson, Missouri, I headed south to the little town of Lincoln, Arkansas, to spend some time visiting with my friend Bud, aka Brutus Knuckles. Bud introduced me to his longtime friend Rory Stockton, who is quite the historian, knowledgeable of many historical events that have taken place in those parts of the country. Rory was kind enough to drive Bud and me around the area one day during my visit and tell us about a hard-fought battle that involved a heated skirmish between the north and the south during the Civil War. I learned that a lot of soldiers died during the fierce battle in the area. Later on, Rory took Bud and me to a drive-in fast-food place called Sonic for a bite to eat.

On a separate occasion, Bud took me to an old cemetery, where there were slaves who lived and died in the area. There is also a marker inscribed with the name of a man who settled in the area with his family. He was a veteran of the Revolutionary War. The individual slave grave sites have a solitary rock that was used to mark the sight, with no names written on it, where each slave was laid to rest. Bud said, "There were also a lot of white people who, when they died, had an unmarked rock placed at the head of the grave."

On another day, Bud drove me to an old cemetery a number of miles from Lincoln to spend time looking at old tombstones, where the names of people are marked with old birth dates and the date they died. There was a small creek flowing nearby the cemetery that sunny April spring day, and Bud and I had a good time being together again, looking at the historical cemetery's tombstones of people long forgotten by many in this ever-busy world. Bud shared with me that the very first church built in Washington County in 1824 was right next to where the cemetery is today. Bud also told me, "There is a bronze plaque marking where the cemetery is and where the former church stood behind the plaque," and he shared the quote on the plaque.

After having a five-day visit with my good friend Bud, I left Lincoln, Arkansas, and drove west to Tulsa, Oklahoma, to see Oral Roberts University. I was able to see the giant praying hands as you enter the university campus. I observed the prayer tower, where hurting people's prayer requests are prayed over on a daily basis year-round. God has answered Christians' prayer needs with amazing miracles down through the years as His people ask and believe Him for great things.

From Tulsa, I drove south on Highway I-44 to Oklahoma City to see where the federal building had been bombed, killing 168 innocent people. The walls surrounding the federal building have been turned into a memorial honoring the people who died there, and now there are flowers, American flags, and pictures of fallen heroes. Inside the walls has been turned into a cemetery, with tombstone markers for the ones who lost their lives inside the federal building. The sad news of the bombing by those associated with the act of terrorism sobered America up to the reality of terrorism in its most evil form in our homeland as well as on foreign soil. Real people are killed by malicious and ruthless villains and taken from us violently, which is pure evil.

When I left Oklahoma City, I headed west on I-40 continuing through Oklahoma and right through the Texas Panhandle. I stayed on Highway I-40 into New Mexico, where I decided to hold up for the night at a rest area. During the day, I continued driving west until I reached Albuquerque, New Mexico, where I drove around parts of the city to see the area—that way I would be able to say that I had been there. After leaving Albuquerque, I kept driving west on I-40 right through New Mexico and directly into the state of Arizona.

I appreciated each state of the union I drove through, with their unique characteristics of national pride and unique qualities of scenic beauty. I saw the sign to the Grand Canyon, but I continued my travels onward until I passed Hoover Dam on my way into Las Vegas, Nevada. There I drove around the big city for a while, held up in one of the park's parking lot for a good part of the day, and ended up seeing the city of Las Vegas at night, with all of its tinsel and glitter from the dazzling lights of entertainment centers. Las Vegas is a showcase of entertainment, with live shows during the day and into the night, as well as a host of gambling casinos, which attract millions each year.

I drove around Las Vegas looking for the establishment my nephew Travis worked at. I had discovered that during his stay in Las Vegas, he has met a lot of famous celebrities. I never found my nephew that night, and I never did go to any of the places of entertainment during my stopover in Vegas. My lovely wife, Lorena, and I flew to Las Vegas as a married couple on a separate minivacation one November day. We enjoyed the sights of entertainment with some of Lorena's family members.

After leaving Las Vegas, I traveled south on Highway 15, and then I took 127 north into Death Valley, where many souls never survived their experience nor lived through their encounter with its desert heat. I wanted to see Death Valley for myself, including the land with its varied terrain that had attracted unsuspecting visitors, some of whom never came out alive. Although I had an excellent rental car with a good air-conditioner, I was mindful that this area can get really hot during the rising temperatures and especially during the summer months.

I drove for some distance into the desert before I stopped to use a pay phone to call the Scone family home in Clover Valley. No one else was at the pull-off stop when I called home that spring day. I told my mother, Jessica, where I was, and she was somewhat surprised that I would be there of all places in the United States. When I hung up from talking to Jessica, she called her daughter Marlie in southern Idaho, and told her where I was. Marlie had heard that day on the news that the hottest place in America that day was Death Valley.

I continued my drive through Death Valley; I didn't experience a lot of vehicle traffic in the desert region that day. I pulled into the visitor center to check it out. Inside the center, I learned that every year one or two people die in Death Valley. I also heard about a honeymoon couple where the husband decided he wanted to walk across the desert. The husband made the long hike across the desert to the mountain range, and on his way back, he expired and died shortly before reaching the road where their car was parked. I also learned about an older gentleman who walked out on the sand dunes in the desert and expired in the desert heat.

The people who do not survive the extreme desert temperatures are not properly equipped to deal with the dry, sandy region with unrelenting and intense heat. The sun beats down on the unprotected head of the desert traveler. It's best to always wear a hat and bring plenty of water whenever you might take a long hike—or even a short walk-in Death Valley. Be well prepared to protect yourself from its extreme elements, which you would not normally deal with on a walk in the woods.

I was perceptive of the other visitors, who would look over at me as I talked to the representatives at the visitor center. I was well aware that the general public would look at me with certain looks that gave me the impression they didn't like what they were looking at or that they had a problem with my physical appearance. I knew that misdirected cosmetic surgeries had left me with an unusual physical appearance that didn't cause people to look at me with pleasant smiles on their faces. I was dealt a cruel hand of unpleasant cosmetic surgeries, which I was left to deal with on a daily basis.

When I pulled out from the Death Valley Visitor Center, I continued my drive through the Death Valley National Park. I drove to the area where the sand dunes were and pulled over to the side of the road. I got out of my rental car, and off in the distance, I could see three hikers on their way back to the main road where I was parked. I also could see two hikers walking across the sand dunes away from me toward the west side of the valley. I took time to try to catch some lizards, which with amazing quickness and speed darted among the wild desert sagebrush. I came awfully close to getting hold of the long tail of one of the desert speedsters, but when I was ready to pinch the end of its tail between my right thumb and index finger, it suddenly darted off to safety among the desert thicket.

After experiencing a portion of the dunes, I headed back to my rental car and continued driving through the national park. I saw the signs for Furnace Creek and Ghost Town, but I decided to continue my drive through the desert valley and head north to Reno, Nevada. I drove through Carson City and Virginia City and made the drive up to beautiful Lake Tahoe. I also saw the sign for the Ponderosa Ranch, a theme park based on the fictionalized television series *Bonanza*. I was told by a staff member of an environmental agency that it is seventy-five miles and approximately an hour and a half from Lake Tahoe. I drove around the lake and held up in a private park, where I took it easy and relaxed for hours in my vehicle. At one point, I got out of the car and walked over to take a look at the beautiful lake waters from the sandy beach viewpoint.

I took notice of certain individuals wondering what I was doing in their private neighborhood park, but I tried not to take it personally by making a quick exit. I eventually drove out from the parking lot. I headed north to see the city of Reno on a beautiful spring night. Again, I never went into any of Reno's entertainment centers, but I could see certain people inside and I knew the gambling casinos had their usual crowd of players seeking their luck, wishing they could win the jackpot and score by beating the house odds. I have learned from experience that most people end up with fool's gold of bad luck and go home poorer than when they entered the casino in the first place with the hope of striking it rich.

After driving around Reno, Nevada for a while and seeing the sights, I drove southwest to I-80 toward Sacramento, California. When I saw the sign for I-5 north, I continued my journey toward home in the Pacific Northwest. I stopped for gas whenever I needed to and for a bite to eat at a fast-food joint when I was hungry. I was determined to drive at night and throughout the day unless I physically couldn't continue on without getting some sleep on my lengthy trip home. I was determined to get home, where I could relax in my own bed and hide out in isolation from the scrutinizing eyes of unfriendly people.

I drove through the northern part of California and through the state of Oregon on I-5. I eventually made it home, where I reside south of Union, without an incident of unfortunate circumstances, which I could have encountered during my cross-country, marathon journey. God protected me from harm on my solo cross-country trip in a lone rental car and gave me safe traveling mercies to reach my home in a quiet residential neighborhood.

I finally met a lovely lady named Lorena Gonzalez, whom I asked to marry me after a long courtship. I knew I'd better not let this beautiful woman who was willing to marry me get away. I met Lorena on one of my William County personnel carrier routes one night while I was waiting until it was time to start my carrier route. Not knowing who this jet-black-haired beauty was, I opened the door of my carrier coach. In walked an attractive woman who sat down across from me; I was sitting in my driver's seat.

The lovely lady inquired if I was going to be leaving soon. I answered her in the affirmative, and I asked her where she was from because of her accent. She responded, Colombia, in a spirited manner. I responded, "Como estas?" in my limited Spanish; I should have said, "Como esta usted?" The Spanish lady told me that she was fine. We continued talking together, and when it became time to leave on my next trip, I said, "Andale! Andale!" which means hurry up in Spanish. The sweet Latina lady told me that *andale* is used by Mexican Spanish-speaking people, whereas *rapido* is used by Spanish-speaking people for the word hurry. I found out that *rapido* can be used for quick, fast, or hurry up. As Lorena was getting off my bus, she said, "Bye." I responded to her, "Buenas noches" for good night.

THE ULTIMATE VIOLATION

The third time that Lorena came onto my personnel carrier, she gave me a Spanish-English dictionary to improve my Spanish vocabulary. On the inside of the cover, she wrote me a nice note, which read, "Kurtess: If you have any questions about Spanish, you can call me at . . ." She included her phone number for me to call. She signed it, "Lorena," with the date included.

Lorena mentioned that maybe we could get together sometime for lunch or for coffee. I contacted Lorena at the phone number she left with me, and we had a good talk in spite of her limited English and my limited Spanish. I told Lorena that I was seeing someone at the time, and so we decided not to pursue a relationship with each other at that time.

Three years later, when I found that my friendship with my lady friend wasn't heading toward marriage, I called and left a message on Lorena's answering machine, saying, "Feliz Navidad and Feliz Ano Nuevo." I didn't know if she was still living at the same place, or even still living in Union.

When Lorena heard the friendly message I had left for her on the recorder, she called me on the phone. We talked on the phone for a couple of weeks before we decided to get together and talk. By now, Lorena spoke much better English, but I hadn't improved much on my Spanish. I discovered that Lorena came from a family of traditional religious beliefs, which she observed growing up in Bogota, Colombia, in South America. Lorena wanted to learn more about God while living in the United States, and I found myself sharing the wonderful truths of Jesus Christ and His free gift of salvation with Lorena.

Lorena had seen Christians on television preaching and sharing about the power of God with their viewing audience. Lorena had even witnessed the power of God being manifested in the lives of the Christian people through the pictures she observed electronically transmitted through the airwaves directly into her apartment living room. Lorena wanted to experience that same power for herself, but she found herself living her life desiring after something that seemed to be elusive from her own existence.

One day I happened to pray for Lorena for the Holy Spirit to touch her life and show Himself mighty on her behalf. I prayed with power as I laid my hands on her head in earnest prayer. The Holy Spirit manifested Himself to Lorena in a special way while she knelt in prayer, and she went limp, as if she were silently fainting in the Lord's presence. Each time I

237

prayed with heartfelt intensity for the power of God Almighty, the Holy Spirit, which is the Spirit of Christ, to manifest Himself to Lorena in His own special way and with power, she experienced the same wonderful touch of the Lord. Lorena discovered the wonderful power of the Lord gloriously manifested on and in her life that special night. Lorena now wanted to become a born-again Christian and to live her life for Christ Jesus as observed in the Christian faith. Lorena discovered God's truths for a godly Christian life were revealed in the Holy Bible to live by, not according to the traditions observed in her traditional South American church.

The Lord has been faithful to Lorena and me. We were married at the Union Covenant Church. We went to Kauai, which is an island of Hawaii, for our honeymoon. Our departure flight from the SeaTac International Airport to Hawaii Island was long, but our flight took place on a beautiful spring day. When we arrived at the very nice resort in Kauai, we decided to go for the upgrade, which was a deluxe hotel suite, which we enjoyed together. Unfortunately the weather wasn't as conducive for outdoor activities as we would have liked during our maiden voyage as a married couple; on honeymoons, you would like to have the most perfect, memorable experience with your spouse.

Lorena and I never went into the Pacific Ocean waters during our honeymoon because of the windy conditions and the rough waters; we didn't want to have any disasters while on our honeymoon. I remember listening to the news in our deluxe hotel room and hearing about the possibility of a tsunami heading toward the Hawaii Islands, which never happened, thank goodness. I didn't want a hundred-foot wall of water slamming into our hotel suite during our stay. Just hearing about the scary chance of having a tsunami looming in a threatening way to destroy our pleasant vacation was not an enjoyable thought.

Lorena and I drove around wanting to take in the scenery we could experience on the garden island in all of its tropical beauty. We went to one beach on a windy day, and we were able to go shopping on a number of occasions together. For Lorena and me, just being together on our first vacation as husband and wife was well worth the honeymoon trip. I decided to go to Kauai out of all of the Hawaiian Islands to avoid the crowds on the other islands and to have the opportunity to get to know one another in romantic solitude. The good Lord provided Lorena and me with a wonderful honeymoon, and when it came time to leave the tropical garden island, we flew home to the Pacific Northwest to continue growing, working on, and experiencing our married life together.

Lorena and I flew down to Las Vegas, Nevada, one year to join Lorena's family members Cecilia, Jose, Carlos, and Ugo Gonzalez. For fun, I decided to make an announcement to the family with my lovely wife present in a hotel room. I spoke in Spanish, which is their native tongue, so they would get the full impact of the message shared. When I had the floor to say something, I took full advantage of the serene moment. With all eyes looking in my direction, I said, "Mi familia. Mi feliz esposa. Estaba virgin," which translates as, "My family. My happy wife. She was a virgin." We all had a good laugh together over my announcement spoken in jest. Lorena and I had a good time together as a married couple and also with my wife's family during our stay. Unfortunately for Lorena and me, we ended up leaving Las Vegas poorer than when we had initially arrived in the entertainment city due to losing at the slot machines. I was able to enjoy myself during our miniature vacation getaway. I was still self-conscious about my physical appearance, but the vacation helped to divert my attention from my outward appearance to marital and family values and being involved in outside and indoor activities.

When Lorena and I visited her family in Bogota, Colombia, in 2007, we witnessed the people of Colombia protesting the long struggle with the guerillas. The people were carrying white flags and honking their car horns throughout Bogota, the capital city of the South American country. They were longing for peace in all of Colombia, and they were tired of the fighting between the democratic Colombian government and the guerilla rebel groups. I wanted to videotape the historic moment of seeing the large groups of Colombians out in force demonstrating their hearts' desire for a peaceful resolution to the evil atrocities and the conflicts of war with the rebels. Unfortunately I discovered I had left behind my battery pack at my sister-in-law Cecilia Gonzalez's apartment. I was disappointed that I had missed out on recording the historic moment.

When Lorena and I were in Bogota in 2007, Margarita Romero, a friend of my sister-in-law Melony Garcia, asked for me to pray for her son John. I anointed John's body with oil, and I prayed the prayer of faith over him. As a positive result, God healed John, and he was feeling better afterward. In 2009, Margarita called Lorena in North America requesting that I pray for John's heart to be healed. John was facing the possibility of open-heart surgery, and he needed a miracle healing touch from the

Master's hand. I prayed over the phone for John's heart to be healed and to be made whole. I prayed that Jesus Christ, who is the same today, yesterday, and forever, to reach down His healing hand of virtue and heal John from the top of his head to the soles of his feet. The latest I heard concerning John's heart condition is that his heart is doing just fine. I know that I am only a vessel through whom God has worked when I have prayed for people and that Jesus is the Healer. I could not heal a flea with a migraine headache, but Jesus is perfectly able to heal all those who call upon His blessed name believing in faith. All the glory belongs to Jesus Christ.

Margarita Romero invited Lorena and me to have lunch with her and her son John while we were in Bogota, Colombia, in 2009. She shared with us that she had seen Pastor Alvarez while watching television, and she discovered during an advertisement where he was going to be speaking when he was in Bogota. Margarita went to the Christian church where he was ministering to the people, and she went up for special prayer concerning herself. Margarita gave a check to his ministry, and she told him she would like to talk to him. He asked her to wait outside of the church for him. Later on, Pastor Alvarez came outside to give Margarita his Miami, Florida, cell number; and when he was back in Miami, she called the number he had given to her. The man of God prayed for her over the phone to be blessed and prosperous, and as a benefit of his prayers for her to be blessed, she had faith to believe God would make provision for her to buy a beautiful apartment where she and her son now live. She also shared that she had purchased a car too. The Lord adds His blessings beyond measure in ways that are best for His people. He only asks for us to believe in Him for a harvest of souls and what we need in life, expect in faith, and when we give tithes and offerings unto the Lord to be cheerful givers.

Lorena informed me that her nephew Denton Garcia wanted to sell his grandfather's stamp collection. Melony Garcia, Denton's mother, brought the extensive stamp collection with her when she came up for Lorena's and my wedding, and Lorena stored the collection in our master bedroom's closet. I heard that Denton wanted to see about selling the stamps, but I wasn't aware that they were sitting up on a shelf in our closet upstairs. Lorena was waiting for Denton to come to the United States so that I could help her nephew sell the collection for whatever it was worth and hopefully come into some good money. Denton told Lorena when we

240

were in Bogota, Colombia, to go ahead and sell the stamp collection and give him whatever she wanted to.

When I became aware of the stamp collection that had been sitting on the closet shelf in our bedroom, I began to think that the collection as a whole was possibly worth thousands if not millions of dollars. Lorena began to think that we now were going to be able to pay off our credit cards and she would be able to buy some things that she wanted and needed for herself. Lorena and I began to look at the dates of some of the stamps, which were well organized in a large book designed for a stamp collection. It was obvious that Denton's grandfather had spent a lot of time on his hobby of collecting foreign, US, and Vatican stamps, both used and unused. I was convinced that this eclectic collection of stamps, if sold at an auction or sold to certain stamp investors, would bring in millions of dollars. The possibilities raised our hopes with lofty dreams of becoming rich, able to retire, enjoy a leisurely life of Riley, and travel whenever and wherever. I thought we were going to be rich after selling the stamps, so I made certain I kept the stamps in the same sack she had originally placed them in and I kept them in our bedroom where I slept to protect the stamps' safety.

On the day that Lorena and I had decided to take the stamp collection for an appraisal, she had a doctor's appointment. I made sure I had the stamp collection with us when I drove Lorena to her doctor's appointment. I didn't even leave the stamps in our car while parked in a parking garage during Lorena's appointment. I thought I was carrying a fortune.

When Lorena and I went to a stamp collection store in Canton to see if the historical stamps had any real value, I was informed by Jeff Thurman, who looked through the large book containing the numerous old stamps, that they had been damaged by the way they were handled. Lorena and I learned the cold hard truth that day that Denton's grandfather, who had taken the time to place them in the book well enough, had used white tape on the underside of each stamp. By doing so, he damaged the stamps so that they lost their true monetary value. The serious reality in hearing the disappointing news from Jeff about the devalued stamps caused Lorena and me to forget about any hopes for any future fortune we had hoped for.

Without taking any more time, Jeff concluded that he wasn't interested in examining any more of the stamps, which were also inside a lot of envelopes, and he wasn't interested in purchasing the damaged collection, although many of the stamps seemed to have historical value to novice stamp collectors. Lorena and I drove out to Rowen to have a second opinion concerning the stamp collection's possible value. Once again, we received news that the store was not interested in buying what we had to sell. For all of our efforts, I was able to sell three Reichmark bank notes for a total of one dollar and one South Korea ten dollar bill for two dollars to a coin collection store in Keeler.

It truly had not turned out to be a profitable day for selling things for Lorena and me, but at least we had satisfied our curiosity for the time being. I thought about going through the old stamp collection at our home just to see if perhaps the professional stamp collection experts might have missed something by not taking the time to examine the entire collection. So far, I never have taken the time to do so, but I hope some rare stamps might be hidden in the mix and not damaged by the beginner stamp collector, who had collected the stamps just for a hobby and possibly not even thought about giving them to any of his descendants on a fine day.

I recognize that just as stamps and coins can be rejected due to physical damages caused because they have been improperly handled, so real people can also experience undue hardships in life because of improper training in medical and cosmetic specialties.

My wife, Lorena, thinks that I would need to look like a monster for me to write my own book. I know that my wife loves me and she hasn't gone through all the unnecessary suffering that I have undergone mentally, emotionally, socially, and physically to fully understand the need for me to write a book on medical malpractice from my perspective. Innocent patients are being hurt by unqualified medical doctors who are driven by power and greed to perform unnecessary cosmetic changes, which result in cosmetic physical violations.

When Lorena looks at her husband's nose, she perceives his physical characteristics in her evaluation as perfect and now down from its previous elevated position where Dr. Cutter placed it against God's creative cosmetic blueprint for me. I recognize the superior skills of a certified American Board of Plastic Surgery surgeon who has performed reconstruction revisions to my damaged physical characteristics. I can still see a noticeable gap between my nose and the outline of the top of my mustache, where Dr. Rockwell worked surgically to bring my nose back down. I also continuously observe the residual longterm consequences and effects of Dr. Cutter's contrary, adverse, and botched surgical work on my nose and ears when I look in the mirror regardless of Dr. Rockwell's corrective revisions and surgical efforts at repair.

I recall the first thing that Dr. Rockwell said to me when I initially came in to see him for an office visit. Dr. Rockwell did not say, "It's nice to see you, Mr. Scone. My name is Dr. Rockwell. How can I be of help to you?" Instead, Dr. Rockwell said to me, "You're not bringing it down," referring to my elevated nose position caused by Dr. Cutter. I have had to pay through the nose in more ways than one.

When Lorena and I flew into the El Dorado airport in Bogota, Colombia, in 2007, a large number of Lorena's wonderful family members were waiting for us. Due to heightened security, all those looking for their family and friends anxiously waited on the outside of the airport for their loved ones to come out of the building. Lorena and I were like celebrities from America, with adoring fans peering in through the windows of the airport hoping to catch a glimpse of the special married couple, who were received as romantic stars from a distant land.

I had brought my music horn, battery-operated speaker along on the trip to greet my new Colombian family with. Once outside of the airport, where Lorena's family were eagerly waiting, for fun I spoke through the speaker to my loving Colombian family by saying, "Hola, Familia. Pancho Villa aqui en Bogota, Colombia," which translated into English means, "Hello family. Pancho Villa is in Bogota, Colombia."

Lorena and I provided all of the stardom status to the family, who were incredibly accepting, warm, kind, loving, generous, inviting, and hospitable in every way to Lorena and me during our two-month stay in Colombia. While visiting with our family, Lorena and I went to Santa Martha, Cartegena, and San Andres with Papi Octavio Gonzalez and Cecilia Gonzalez, Kurtess's father-in-law and sister-in-law. The four of us had a good time each time we went on a minivacation getaway to the Colombian resorts in the summer of 2007.

I have come to love and appreciate my Colombian family because they are such loving, accepting, kindhearted, generous, and hospitable people. They are truly precious people, who have made me feel loved, admired, and accepted as part of their extended family. I thank the Lord Jesus for all of my close Colombian family.

Lorena and I went to an all-boys orphanage with our Colombian family when visiting Bogota. Lorena and I wanted to make a difference in the lives of the boys living at the home by providing shoes for them. Lorena's brother Jaime made a special contribution to the boys, with clothing items they could use such as underwear and socks. For Lorena and me, it was a first-time experience of actually going to and being at an orphanage.

I found that I enjoyed the good foods, fruits, and variety of tasty and healthy juice drinks Colombia has to offer. I discovered that I appreciated churrasco and carne asada, which are Colombian steaks served at the restaurants or enjoyed at a family member's home. I also enjoyed the various soups like Santafereno, and healthy salads. I experienced huevos like eggs a la cazuela. I also enjoyed many tropical fruits that are common to the country, Colombian candies, Colombian coffee, and delicious juices, which helped to reduce the sugars in my diet.

Lorena and I enjoyed our visits to Colombia in 2007 and in 2009. The one negative thing was the extremely fast driving by taxi drivers, whose driving in traffic can be a scary experience for a foreigner to their country. I thank Dios (God) that Lorena and I were never involved in an accident during our numerous rides in taxis while visiting Colombia. There are some travelers who are not as lucky.

Lorena and I both opted to have surgery with Dr. Raymond Rockwell in Los Angeles. It would be Lorena's first time to have any surgeries with Dr. Rockwell. I decided to have a chin revision in hopes to have my left side evenly matched up with the right side of my chin. Dr. Rockwell's surgical procedure included placing a plastic device under the left side of my chin area to augment my chin to look more evenly balanced in appearance with the right side. My chin swelled up postsurgery due to the surgical procedure, and I hoped the swelling would disappear before Lorena and I left for Bogota, Colombia. Unfortunately not all of the swelling in my chin had subsided within the two-and-a-half-month postsurgery span of time. The object inserted under my chin covered a portion under my left jaw area and gave the unsightly appearance of a protruding tumor.

During the three-week vacation to Colombia, Lorena told me that family members and friends of the family were wondering what I had inside of my good-looking face. Lorena informed everyone in Bogota that was questioning my unpleasant appearance that a medical doctor had placed it there and he was going to remove it when I went back home. It was not my cosmetic interest to have a protruding device appearing under one side of my chin area to provide me with an evenly balanced chin. Lorena agreed with me that I should have the necessary corrective surgery by Dr. Rockwell to remove the hard plastic device made of silicone that he had put under my chin area.

Dr. Rockwell had mentioned to me that he couldn't figure out why my first doctor had put screws in my chin since it was a routine chin implant. When I initially thought on the matter, I couldn't recall ever having Dr. Smith or Dr. Cutter mention putting screws into my jaw for any medical or cosmetic reason. I began to suspect that Dr. Cutter had possibly put the screws into my jaw as a way to let me know that I had been screwed by the malicious medical doctor. I knew that Dr. Thadeaus Damon Cutter had truly victimized me, but I was not in a position to say that Dr. Cutter was the doctor who had placed the screws into my chin.

Later, when I decided to pursue my quest for a valid answer to my nagging suspicions concerning Dr. Cutter, Dr. Rockwell provided me a more logical explanation to put my inquisitive mind to rest. Dr. Rockwell informed me that he didn't have the old preop reports regarding my chin implant so he didn't know who had done the procedure. But he knew that whoever did the first chin implant would have broken the chinbone to slide it forward, an osteotomy, and then would have put in a screw to hold it in place.

Dr. Rockwell's explanation made perfect sense to me regarding the medical procedure on my chin, but I had been hoping to hear that he suspected the second doctor put the screw or screws in place; that would have clearly pointed back to Dr. Cutter as the real culprit. I recognize that I had good reason to suspect Dr. Cutter with fraud regarding my chin along with the work in concert on my nose and ears, but I was willing to listen to a cosmetic expert who knew the procedures and medical terms.

I was able to locate the preop report at home, and I sent a copy to Dr. Rockwell. Dr. Rockwell now had the preop report as evidence that Dr. Cutter put the screws in my chin. Dr. Rockwell now had the evidence in his possession that I had wondered about, which showed that Dr. Cutter had been the medical doctor who put the screws into my chin. I thought to myself that I had been literally screwed by Dr. Cutter, and I took it in the chin.

I was able to find Dr. Cutter's release of records, including an operation report for me. I read, "Once the horizontal cut had been completed, the chin distal fragment was advanced forward. An Osteomed bone plate using a 10 mm chin plate was adapted to create a 9 mm advancement graft of the chin and secured with four 6 mm screws. Care was taken to keep the midline in the correct position." I planned to send the operation report to Dr. Raymond Rockwell for his own medical information. For me, this was verification that Dr. Cutter had put the screws into my chin; I had read about it in Dr. Cutter's medical operation report.

I discovered firsthand that history has a way of repeating itself. When I reflect back to my hitting experience as a teenager against a future major league baseball pitcher named Gary Holland, even though I recall seeing a white streak quickly hurtling toward me, for me it was like a blind man looking for a black cat in a dark room. To me, with Dr. Cutter it was a repeat of not beating the competition. I at the time did not even know I was competing with Dr. Cutter. My cosmetic experience with Dr. Cutter, a nonspecialized medical doctor in the nose and ears, once again was like a blind man looking for a black cat in a dark room.

No unsuspecting patient wants to go through the horrifying cosmetic experience that I have undergone, and I dare to say not even Dr. Cutter himself would. I am convinced that even Dr. Cutter, with the conniving approach that he took against me, knew full well that he had painfully hurt an innocent cosmetic patient because he didn't have the specialized training that was necessary. Going by Dr. Cutter's actions pre- and postsurgery, I know that Dr. Cutter woke up to actually observe for himself the unqualified surgical damages that he had inflicted on my nose and ears. For this reason, I know beyond a shadow of a doubt that Dr. Cutter didn't try to contend with the licensing boards to continue practicing cosmetic surgeries on patients who had more than one surgery on their nose and ears.

If Dr. Cutter would volunteer to have a cosmetic surgeon with a general in cosmetic surgery and a secondary in plastic surgery cosmetically work on his nose and ears after he had undergone numerous surgeries on his nose and ears, would he consider that equal treatment and being fair-handed for what I underwent postsurgery? Or would he consider facing a nonspecialized cosmetic surgeon after having multiple surgeries on his physical characteristics an unfair deal, and a more accurate description of cosmetic crimes of a deranged, delusional, and psychotic type of a medical doctor? I am persuaded that Dr. Cutter expected for me to be delusional in my postsurgery thinking and believed that he could control a subdued subject that was mentally not all there. Dr. Cutter discovered to his surprise that I still had certain mental faculties remaining that came back to haunt him in his cosmetic practice. I am convinced that Dr. Cutter decided to move from Victimized, USA, to Victimization, USA, because of trying to distance himself from his cosmetic crimes that he committed against me and other unsuspecting patients. He has made victims out of his patients, and he covers it up by putting distance between him and his victims.

I recognize that there is a day of reckoning coming for every power-tripping medical doctor willing to abuse, exploit, and victimize unsuspecting cosmetic patients, if not in this world, then on Judgment Day when they meet God as their judge.

To the above, I say, "Let justice prevail."

I recall sending in my first series of complaints to the different medical boards Dr. Cutter was licensed with. I remember saying in my first complaint letter that I was trusting that Dr. Cutter could do what I cosmetically wanted for him to do, which was absolutely not the case at all. I was so horribly traumatized, painfully devastated, and agonizingly cosmetically violated that when it came to sending in my complaints over a number of years after surgery, I still hadn't fully comprehended the total magnitude of Dr. Cutter's incalculable damages to my total man. I have come to the realization that Dr. Cutter completely took out any trust from my soul when he boldly took charge of my cosmetic destiny without my consent nor partial or full understanding, and helped himself to my nose and ears, for which he had positively no specialization. It has become a long, painful process for me to exist in a world where people are judged on the basis of whether they physically meet the world's standards of acceptance, approval, and success.

I contacted Arnold Richards, chief investigator of MQAC, and inquired if I could find out how long the medical board and the investigator unit had kept my case open against Dr. Cutter. I inquired how I could find that information, and he told me that it went to the archives of the state. Arnold informed me that I could find that information through public disclosure. I cordially thanked him and hung up the phone. I waited a short while and called back, hoping to find out the information I was pursuing from another representative over the phone. The woman who answered the phone on my next call transferred me to another female representative, who in turn transferred me to Arnold, chief investigator. Arnold let me know in no uncertain terms that he had already told me what I needed to do. He told me again that I could find the information through public disclosure. He told me he didn't want me to be talking to his staff trying to find the information I was wanting. He let me know they had already been told not to respond to me. He told me they were willing to work with me, but I needed to find out what I was looking for through public disclosure.

By the sound of Arnold's corrective, determined tone of voice, I had pushed his buttons by talking to his staff. I did not know I was talking to Arnold's female staff members when I called back to acquire the information I wanted over the phone instead of waiting for some personnel of the state to search for my files now in the archives of the state. By the corrective rebuke I received from Arnold over the phone, it's obvious to me that I have made a nuisance out of myself by calling far too many times to the MQAC over the years pursuing a decisive judgment. I also recognize that I was suffering from postsurgery trauma for years resulting from Dr. Cutters actions initiated against me. Arnold answered me by inferring the information I was seeking was not there, but at a different location, the archives of the state. I know I didn't need Arnold's overbearing, irritated, authoritarian attitude as a representative of the state when I called back wanting to get information over the phone regarding my case against Dr. Cutter. I was not being pushy in my endeavors with any representative I spoke with. I realize the emphasis should not be on me being persistent about finding answers, but upon their losing patience with me and how they failed to take corrective action against Dr. Cutter. My persistence over the years was prompted by their lack of action against the sinister medical doctor. By Arnold's attitude, he showed me that he and his staff do not care about people in my predicament. I thanked Arnold the second time and hung up the phone.

I know for an absolute fact that Dr. Cutter committed crimes against me not based upon a sad case of hypochondria, mere speculation, or a whole lot of guesswork, but based upon experiential knowledge, Dr. Cutter's own admission, eyewitness accounts, negatively impacting, hard-hitting experiences, and hard reality evidence. I came to realize that God knows, the devil knows, Dr. Cutter knows, and I came to know that Dr. Cutter had committed medical malpractice crimes against me. And now the whole wide world knows that the Dr. Cutters of this world, by their own track records, consistently violate and victimize unsuspecting cosmetic patients.

I have discovered that, just as in the bird or animal kingdoms, if there is one that is viewed as being weak, odd, strange, or abnormal, it can expect to be picked on or rejected by the rest of the group. The teachings of psychology and evolution agree with this, because they promote it. But God's Word is very clear that the problem abides in the fallen human nature that began in the Garden of Eden. I have experienced the coldness of social rejections by the general public, and I am convinced that was largely caused by the cruel, criminal, and immoral actions of a malicious cosmetic surgeon disguised as a medical doctor.

Dr. Cutter wanted to express the desires of the god of this world's fallen system toward my facial characteristics according to his own specifications and prove to me and the general public that he could tear down and rebuild my physical features to my original specifications as detailed in my postsurgery desired results notes, which the cosmetic surgeon copied for himself.

The god of this world's system is the devil, according to the Holy Bible, and I have come to the realization of how Dr. Cutter committed his crimes against me on the day of my surgeries. I was talking to my counselor Norman Dodson, and he shared with me how he learned to conduct instant hypnotism on another person while in his counseling training. I knew that I wasn't delusional in my thinking about what I had experienced at the hands of Dr. Cutter.

I had wondered for years why a medical doctor would move out of his specialization of dentistry and cosmetically work on my nose and ears without any specialization in the nose and ears. Dr. Cutter was so narcissistically in love with himself that he wanted to play God with my facial characteristics; it started as a fantasy in his mind, and ended up as a horrible cosmetic travesty for his subdued subject.

I came to the realization the reason why Dr. Cutter hadn't connected with me pre- and postsurgery was for him to play cosmetic fantasy with my physical characteristics. Law officials will acknowledge that many crimes start out as a fantasy in the minds of the criminal and then are acted out in reality in real-life situations that end in the victimization of an unsuspecting person. This explains why I didn't have any understanding of Dr. Cutter's change in cosmetic plans on the day of my surgeries and why I heard Dr. Cutter say while I was coming to when I was still on the operating table, "You're going to like it."

I recall the last thing I thought about before blanking out on the day of my surgeries was Dr. Cutter saying, "Well, I better go about building up the bridge," referring to the bridge of my nose.

I remember thinking to myself, *Why didn't he tell me this up front?* as I went into unconsciousness.

I am persuaded in my own mind that the reason Dr. Cutter committed his cosmetic and financial crimes against me was to prove to himself, any doctor I might see afterward, and the general public that he could tear down the previous doctors' work on my nose, ears, and chin, and rebuild them to my satisfaction—just as a traumatized victim would be satisfied with the results of a shark attack on his or her amputated or mutilated body part.

Apparently, the review board had to wait for me to come to the realization that I didn't have any understanding of what Dr. Cutter intended on the day of my surgeries back in the nineties to take action against Dr. Cutter.

I know that Dr. Cutter should be included in the United States' and the International Communities' Dumbest Criminals list because he gloated postsurgery about victimizing his cosmetic patient. I realize that loose lips sink ships and had Dr. Cutter been able to come across to me as a caring medical doctor postsurgery, he would have been able to cloak his crimes committed against his patient more deceptively. But Dr. Cutter had a hard time resisting gloating about his victory over his subdued and duped victim by saying, "See it as a sculpture. I tore it down, beat it up, and built it back up."

I never stated in my postsurgery desired results notes, which Dr. Cutter said gave him something to work with, that I wanted for Dr. Cutter to tear down the previous doctors' work and rebuild it all over again, now in an elevated position contrary to my desires. The postsurgery results caused by Dr. Cutter's cosmetic hacking have not gone unnoticed by the general public, which shuns the victim.

I have gone to see my counselor Norman Dodson for a number of years, primarily dealing with the aftermath of my dealings with Dr. Cutter. Norman identified Dr. Cutter as a con artist, similar to a car salesman, who gets slicker and slicker. Norman said, "Since you never encountered that, you didn't know what hit you. Since you're not a con artist, you don't think like a con artist. You have a hard time identifying it. So it really catches you off guard, like a slick car salesman." During one of our counseling sessions, Norman used the word "rape" in reference to Dr. Cutter's actions committed against me.

I could identify with what Norman was describing about my personal experience with Dr. Cutter. I shared with my counselor that I was affected mentally by my experience with Dr. Cutter. Norman questioned me how I had been affected mentally.

I said, "Because I could feel the pressure in my brain." I described to Norman that I felt like I had mental blocks preventing me from remembering certain things that I had experienced. I have come to the realization that the cosmetic plans of Dr. Cutter for his patient were literally shoved up into my brain; they had become elusive to me recollecting memories in detail of what actually happened to me on the day of my surgeries.

Norman said, "You had difficulty retrieving memories."

I recalled hearing Dr. Cutter say while I was coming to on the surgery table, "You're going to like it."

Norman identified those words as mental suggestions given to me by Dr. Cutter.

Presurgery, I remember hearing Dr. Cutter say, "Well, I better go about building up the bridge."

I thought to myself, *Why didn't he tell me this up front?* as my mind went blank.

Norman shared with me that he had learned about performing instant hypnosis on another attendee during an educational training where he had learned about the different forms of hypnosis. They had practiced the technique on each other during the training.

I know that Dr. Cutter utilized hypnosis on me presurgery, and I thereafter experienced irreparable cosmetic damages to my nose and ears.

I remember reading parts of Katharine A. Phillips's book *The Broken Mirror*. The book deals with body dismorphic disorders, whereby people exhibit phobias of not wanting to be visibly seen by other people. They have dreadful, acute feelings of being rejected by others because of their physical appearance. Many people who suffer from this terrible disorder have minor physical flaws, but they avoid human contact because of not wanting to be rejected by some other person for what they physically can't change; they want to hide from being seen by the cynical public, so they will stay at home most of the time.

I am all too aware of this painful phobia, which robs the victims with fears that seek to steal, kill, and destroy a person's relationships with our fellow human beings. I can identify with this horrible disorder, which can hold its victims in an agonizing grip of mental and emotional bondage, with the actions of the cynical judging crowd making them self-conscious and fearful of other people. I have worked at isolating myself from most of the neighbors I have lived around because of not wanting to be seen due to the cosmetic damages caused by Dr. Cutter. I have suffered needlessly in my personal, social, and professional relationships because of the predatory actions of one cosmetic shyster utilizing mental trickery and thuggery on an unsuspecting cosmetic hopeful, who was seeking subtle revision reconstructive work by a board-certified plastic surgeon.

I recall crying as I drove my carrier route out to Fedora Fair with a carrier half full of passengers. My horrible disfigurement inflicted on me by Dr. Cutter, combined with the abusive mental and emotional suffering, had made me reach another breaking point in my life. My devastating experience with the ruthless and malicious cosmetic surgeon was something that I felt like I absolutely didn't need in my life, but I found myself having to deal with the abusive victimization by Dr. Cutter on a daily basis. I would like to have been able to hold back the tears that would roll down my cheeks during my drive, but I found myself reflecting on my unnecessary, hurtful cosmetic experience; and the passengers could clearly see my grief. On this day, I once again was overcome with emotional grief and sadness from the social rejections by the general public, making me feel that I was unacceptable and unlovely although I was accepting, but businesslike to them, when they entered my carrier coach.

I am saddened when I think upon all the victims who are painfully suffering throughout Deception, Victimized, and Victimization, USA, and around the world because of certain medical doctors who are pursuing the pseudo-gods of narcissistic power and greed for filthy lucre.

God's Word says, "For the love of money is the root of all kinds of evil, for which some have strayed from the faith in their greediness, and pierced themselves through with many sorrows" (1 Tim. 6:10).

I have realized that psychotherapy uses hypnosis, and many professionals have learned psychotherapy in part or fully—and utilize it in their various fields of endeavor. I am convinced that Dr. Cutter wanted to see what he could get away with when he decided to pull off his cosmetic heist against me. I am convinced that Dr. Cutter used his cosmetic practice as a surgical weapon to literally deceive me, and the end result proved to me that Dr. Cutter was not a board-certified plastic surgeon, as I wanted and needed. Dr. Cutter showed me by actual demonstration that he could utilize hypnosis on my mind to cosmetically serve up a counterfeit interpretation on my nose and ears.

To me, these actions on the part of Dr. Cutter provided convincing evidence that he was not a plastic surgeon, which I knew I was searching for. Because of his narcissistic tendencies, Dr. Cutter quickly moved me to cosmetic surgeries on my nose, ears, and chin only to force painful, devastating cosmetic changes on my face. Dr. Cutter then forced the plastic surgeon who would perform any revision work on me to make his own professional evaluation as to his cosmetic work being a cosmetic crime or simply a misinterpretation or a misapplication of the surgeon's cosmetic agenda.

I compare a tae kwon do nine grandmaster actually demonstrating on me and my friend Lynn when we wanted only to see a martial arts demonstration as spectators to having Dr. Cutter demonstrating on me. Dr. Cutter demonstrated his cosmetic techniques on me by tearing down the previous doctors' work on my nose and ears and starting from scratch to rebuild them into something that I positively didn't want nor need. I know that Dr. Cutter was a power-tripping, delusional-thinking cosmetic surgeon narcissistically in love with himself to ever dare to endeavor such bold cosmetic procedures on a multiple-surgery patient and as a nonrecognized cosmetic surgeon.

I recognize that it is pathetic to think of all the unsuspecting patients who have been seriously hurt, abused, and victimized by nonrecognized cosmetic surgeons over the years. I know for a 100 percent fact that many of the victimized patients would have self-destructed into the dangers of drugs and alcohol had they gone through what I have had to endure since my surgeries in the nineties. I also recognize that most people would not be able to endure the dangerous waters of social rejections by the general public and the professional rejections by their colleagues at their work environment. Many, sad to say, may resort to suicide with such a disadvantage and being cut out from the good road to successful living.

I wanted to be fair in my evaluation of Dr. Cutter, who never took the time to slow down and properly interpret my cosmetic blueprint from my initial consultation with Dr. Cutter to our third consultation, resulting in my surgeries. I can now see that Dr. Cutter was too obsessed with gaining my cosmetic and financial business to rightly slow down to appropriately interpret precisely what I was wanting and needing of the cosmetic doctor. I am convinced that Dr. Cutter did see the cosmetic light as to what I was wanting and needing cosmetically, but he was too absorbed with demonstrating his own cosmetic agenda, which clashed with what I was desiring.

Dr. Cutter wanted to dislodge, exchange, and replace my cosmetic presurgery images for my nose and ears with his own cosmetic agenda for my physical characteristics. The results were painfully scary for me.

I recommend that health departments, medical boards, and investigators throughout Victimized, USA, not only place a security check against nonrecognized medical professionals, but they need to communicate fully to the victims of medical malpractice verbally and in writing the steps to resolve the tragedy of their victimization so that the victims are fully compensated both physically and financially. To do anything less is to dishonor the very reason that the health departments, medical boards, and investigators exist in the first place. I also recommend that a representative from the above make contact with the victims and personally help the victims by assisting them in making positively certain that they have filled out all the necessary paperwork in order to be fully compensated by the victimizing party.

No longer should the above simply wait until the victims have provided the detailed information should they have the mental recall to remember everything that happened to them and eventually work through their horrible victimization. If there is physical evidence that other medical doctors do not recognize as physically appearing as good, normal, and quality cosmetic results, then there needs to be an immediate criminal investigation by the above-mentioned into the nonrecognized surgeon's practice. The victim should not have to undergo years of counseling or go to psychobabble sessions in order to be financially compensated and have physical damages corrected.

My friend Tommy Ray is a survivor of abuse by an alcoholic father, and he has written a good book entitled *No More*. Tommy has recognized that there are a lot of horrifying abuse cases concerning children going on in the United States, and he has seen the serious need to raise the consciousness level of every public citizen outraged by accusations of abuse and victimization of the little ones growing up in homes throughout our wonderful country blessed by a loving God.

I have talked often with my friend Tommy Ray about the horrible victimization that is taking place in America by nonrecognized medical doctors abusing their positions of trust and victimizing innocent,

THE ULTIMATE VIOLATION

unsuspecting patients with medical malpractice abuses and victimization. Tommy recognizes that from the medical board's position, it would take a lot more than a victimized carrier driver like me to bring down a medical doctor who is one of their own committing cosmetic abuses and cosmetic crimes against the trusting public.

I recognize that I had better have the goods as far as having my facts straight before bringing an accusation against a medical doctor like Dr. Cutter. I am convinced Dr. Cutter committed cosmetic crimes against me. I know for a 100 percent fact that I was victimized by a cosmetic surgeon disguised as a medical doctor. I am a survivor of cosmetic crimes committed against me by a nonrecognized cosmetic surgeon.

I had legitimate fears and concerns that if Dr. Cutter, MD, DDS, seriously victimized and hurt me, if he was not stopped by the medical board and the investigator unit, he would continue to hurt other unsuspecting consumers. I heard my brother Daniel leave a message for me on my answering machine that David Boze, a conservative talk show host on 770 AM, was talking about a medical doctor named Thomas Laney who had lost a patient, and that he was a practicing dentist in Moses Lake, Washington, and a cosmetic surgeon. Daniel knew that I would be interested regarding a case about a medical doctor, MD, and a cosmetic surgeon who had a dental board license, DDS, to practice family dentistry as well, just like Dr. Cutter.

After a commercial break, I was able to hear David share with his listening audience that, "Dr. Laney would have to be a genius, or something wasn't right with him having different boards like that."

David mentioned that there was an article about Dr. Laney in the *Seattle Post Intelligencer* newspaper dated Monday, November 10, 2008. I was able to get a copy of the article on Tuesday, November 11, from a kindhearted passenger since I didn't take the paper myself.

I read the well-written article by P-I reporter Vanessa Ho, which stated the following: "The P-I found that Laney was doing full-body cosmetic surgeries without having done a residency or fellowship in the subject. Instead, Laney trained through sporadic classes. His surgeries led to many malpractice lawsuits and complaints with the state."

I encourage the reader to read the entire article about the lawsuit against the dentist and oral surgeon Dr. Laney, including his botched breast reduction surgery performed on a woman when she was fifteen.

After reading Vanessa's sad report about the woman, who claims Dr. Laney disfigured her during breast surgery, I contacted the Collard library to inquire of the reference librarian if Dr. Laney had been featured in the *Seattle P-I* or the *Seattle Times* before this November 10 newspaper article in the P-I.

The reference librarian referred me to go online to http://www.seattlepi.com/ and type in Dr. Laney under search. As a result, I was able to find another article written by the P-I's investigative reporter Michelle Nicolosi. Her well-written, researched, and informative article tells about the sad story of the death of David Scott Kelley. His death in 2000 was a consequence after he had cosmetic surgery in Dr. Laney's office.

Based upon the above article, I thought it was truly informative that Dr. Laney's training was rather questionable: "Like many practitioners now performing cosmetic surgery, Laney did not get medical school, residency or fellowship training to do many of the cosmetic procedures he now performs."

Dr. Laney was trained as an oral surgeon, completing a dual-degree program that gave him both a medical and a dental degree. For the most part, he said he learned below-the-neck cosmetic surgeries in weekend and weeklong courses held around the country—sometimes in surgical suites and sometimes in hotel rooms, where demonstrations are done on cadavers.

I was particularly fascinated with one paragraph under "Death cases closed quietly," which stated, "Laney said he does have a 'high' number of lawsuits, but said that 'goes with the territory' when you're dealing with patients with high expectations, and with area doctors who are disgruntled that you're working in an arena they consider their territory—doctors who in some cases urged patients to sue. 'Regrettably, litigation is typical and expected in this type of work,' he wrote in a response to questions. Laney said his number of lawsuits is 'near the industry standard.' See Dr. Laney's complete written response."

When I read Dr. Laney's responses to the questions being asked, it gave me the impression that Laney had a cavalier attitude about the high number of lawsuits he had dealt with. To me, Laney's answer clearly revealed that he was in competition with better trained and much more skilled medical doctors in his quest to physically demonstrate that his cosmetic skills were just as qualified as his medical competitors. I could see that Dr. Laney was in competition with better-trained medical doctors. I could clearly see that Dr. Laney's delusional thinking had caused him to forwardly place himself into an arena of surgically victimized, seriously hurting, and devastating, unsuspecting patients' lives. He classifies in my evaluation as a delusional-thinking power tripper and a cosmetic surgeon to be stopped from practicing cosmetic surgeries by the medical board immediately. How many Dr. Laneys and Dr. Cutters is the medical board going to allow to butcher unsuspecting patients?

I recognize that if Dr. Laney is in any way like Dr. Cutter, then the general public is in grave danger of being cosmetically victimized, irreparably physically damaged, and exploited financially. I discovered that the Medical Quality Assurance Commission deals primarily with licensing of medical doctors, and not with medical specialties issues. From my experience with making my complaints known regarding my victimization at the surgical hands of Dr. Cutter, I don't feel that I was taken seriously by the medical review board and the investigator unit.

I understand now that if the medical board doesn't take disciplinary or termination action against a medical doctor within the first two years of someone bringing complaints forward, then you are pleading your case to deaf ears, groups who see things entirely differently than what you believe, realize, recognize, and eventually know for a 100 percent fact. The policies need to be changed to fully protect the patients' care so that there will never be another victim of a medical doctor out to advance his or her professional career and pad his or her financial coffers at the patients' expense. There are real people like me who are being victimized by nonrecognized medical doctors that the medical board and the investigator unit must stop now.

The evidence demands a verdict by the legislators in Olympia, Washington, the Medical Quality Assurance Commission in Olympia, the William County Medical Society in Union, and the Oral Maxillofacial Surgery Commission in Chicago, Illinois, that there is a medical doctor who is mentally delusional on their licensing boards. He is not adequately trained to be doing all the medical cosmetic surgeries as his professional colleagues who are better trained and superior in their medical specialties and have board certification to sufficiently support and back up their surgical skills.

The Dr. Cutters are willing to surgically proceed and practice cutting on unsuspecting patients without having a medical specialty in plastic surgery and reconstructive surgery. This can be very scary for an unsuspecting patient when his cosmetic interests are botched by a medical doctor who led him to believe that the doctor was a medical specialist as an ABMS, and then postsurgery, after he is physically disfigured, he learns that the medical doctor who surgically worked on him was not listed on any one of the twenty-four boards of medical specialties. I recognize that here is clearly a strong case for stricter surgical guidelines of qualified medical surgeons, with excellent judgment of their medical training, surgical skills, and limitations in light of their board or non-board certification status. I recognize that the laws need to be changed to protect the general public by requiring that the medical doctor provide his or her medical history to all his or her patients of every surgery botched due to a lack of medical specialties board certification.

I contacted Patricia Walters at the Medical Quality Assurance Commission, who was the person I needed to go through when I would send in a letter requesting a reconsideration of my closed case by the medical review board against Dr. Cutter. Patricia was the program manager who became acting deputy executive director of the MQAC; she informed me that they had been in the process of moving to a new building and the commission would not be revisiting the issue that the commission closed some time ago. She went on to inform me that it has been a habit for a great deal of time that the commission doesn't review cases for reconsideration after a year or two. Patricia told me that if I had new issues in regard to Dr. Cutter, I could submit the new issues, but for something that happened so long ago, she didn't feel that they would accept my request for a reconsideration at this time. Patricia assured me that the commission had reviewed it thoroughly. She further informed me that she no longer deals with the disciplinary work. She now has a new position with the Medical Quality Assurance Commission. I thought it was particularly interesting that Patricia told me that there were orders based on my previous letters that they were not to respond to me anymore because apparently I had contacted the MQAC far too many times in my quest for answers and wanting them to take action against Dr. Cutter.

I finally received my final letter from Patricia Walters informing me that the commission would not be reopening my case against Dr. Cutter for reconsideration. I was not terribly surprised nor disheartened by the final verdict by the MQAC. I know the medical review board and the investigator unit made a huge mistake when they didn't take disciplinary or termination action against Dr. Cutter in my individual case. I have decided not to send the MQAC any more additional information requesting a reconsideration hearing of my case against Dr. Cutter. I'm going to let them find the additional information in my book *The Ultimate Violation.*

The verdict did not deter me from going forward with my book so that readers may benefit from my troubling victimization. I don't just *believe* I was victimized by Dr. Cutter. I know for a 100 percent fact that I was. I can appreciate that the medical review board heard my second complaint for reconsideration. However, they need to change their policy to allow for the patient to fully figure out what happened to him or her, which may take years, and never close the doors to each hurting patient until they solve each individual case of victimization by a medical doctor—especially if the medical doctor is not recognized by any specialty board, such as the American Board of Plastic Surgery and the American Board of Medical Specialties.

I also contacted Carrie Barkley, who is the current deputy executive director of the MQAC in Olympia. I inquired of Carrie why the MQAC would allow nonrecognized medical doctors to perform surgeries on multiple-surgery patients. I shared with Carrie the story of a medical doctor who advertises as an American Board of Cosmetic Surgery surgeon, which is a made-up board not recognized by the American Board of Plastic Surgery or the American Board of Oral Maxillofacial Surgery. His specialties are in dentistry, I shared with Carrie.

I heard Carrie tell me the same answer that Dr. Cutter's receptionist had given to my coworker Denise years earlier. Carrie said to me, "There are a lot of boards out there." Carrie did not provide me a good explanation why nonrecognized cosmetic surgeons should be recognized as qualified to conduct surgical procedures on multiple-surgery patients.

Carrie wanted to know if I would like to talk to a medical doctor concerning this matter, and I answered, yes.

A short time later, I heard a medical doctor at the Medical Quality Assurance Commission tell me the exact same thing that Carrie had shared with me: "There are a lot of boards out there."

I realize that Dr. Cutter and other nonrecognized medical doctors are exploiting the medical boards' laxity in strict policy guidelines regarding cosmetic procedures on multiple-surgery patients, which should be performed only by Certified American Board Plastic Surgeons. Without a change in policy, surgeries will remain too scary to contemplate for the trusting patients desiring cosmetic work.

I know that I was stonewalled from the beginning regarding my complaints against Dr. Cutter. I did my level best to bring my complaints to the various medical review boards against Dr. Cutter, but I met with cold, apathetic responses from the medical board and the investigator unit reviewing my case. I know I was and am a victim of a multiple-surgery cosmetic bonanza for Dr. Cutter at my expense. I know that it doesn't matter how long my botched surgeries were ignored by the above-mentioned authorities. My complaints against Dr. Cutter should have never been closed, but earnestly pursued until my case was brought to the satisfaction of the victim, Kurtess Lief Scone. I have discovered to my agony that the proper authorities in the medical community are not willing to budge on their complacency when it comes to allowing practice by medical doctors who have other board certifications that are not recognized by the American Board of Plastic Surgery and the American Board of Medical Specialties and these other doctors show by their track records that they do not qualify to be recognized by the specialized boards through proper residency training that they recognize each patient's cosmetic interests with precision, detailed work with superior perfection and excellence. I know that Dr. Cutter had neither board certification, and I know that I was a victim of a malicious medical doctor who took complete advantage of my naïveté when it came to his lack of recognized board certification, which I expected and needed.

I contacted a woman named Beatrice Carlson, a staff member knowledgeable in plastic and cosmetic procedures, who listened patiently to me explain in detail the precarious and dangerous cosmetic ordeal performed on my nose, ears, and chin by Dr. Cutter. I wondered if she could answer my question why the medical boards have not restricted medical doctors from performing multiple-surgery procedures without a board certification from the American Board of Plastic Surgery or the ABMS.

Beatrice gave me a list of good, knowledgeable things someone could use in pursuing the right surgeon for myself or herself. Beatrice didn't feel that she could answer my good question because she recognizes there are different boards that have different requirements, and there are many of them out there that overlap one another and others that don't. You have to do a lot of checking and rechecking, she said. She recognized that you have to ask a lot of specific questions about training, experience, who does the doctor's certification, and how many surgeries the medical doctor you are considering has done. Beatrice recognizes my questions were huge policy questions way beyond the scope of the office she works in, but she thought I could start by contacting the American Board of Medical Specialties. I have already done so.

I heard of a military instructor who has been training soldiers for forty years on how to survive on the battlefield when facing the enemy. I listened intently to the news reporter say that the instructor tells the troops he is training to have faith in God. I was impressed with the leader's advice on how to survive when you're facing full-fledged combat with an enemy that wants to kill you. I want to pass on the same good advice to readers who have experienced hurtful, painful, and devastating cosmetic surgeries, which have been so destructive and a major setback to your dreams of a better-looking, new you and which have led to unforeseen, cosmetic-related physical damages. Have faith in God, and do your very best at remaining positive with supportive, faithful, and loyal friends and family, who love and care about you personally. Look on the bright side of life, and be a positive contributor to all those around you.

I am a survivor of a sinister cosmetic crime, scam, and heist. I have decided that I would like to move from Victimized, USA, to Justification City, USA.

I now realize that encountering the wrong medical doctor is hazardous to your mental, emotional, and physical health. I recognize that corrective cosmetic revisions can be very costly in trying to undo as much as medically and cosmetically possible by the plastic surgeon reconstructionist. For the whole series of corrective revisions to my nose, ears, and chin by Dr. Raymond Rockwell, my total payments came to $24,150.00.

I would be pleased to know that my book, which is based on actual true events, has helped to inform, educate, entertain, and equip the reader to be able to avoid the mistakes and pitfalls that I made in finding the wrong medical doctor and cosmetic surgeon, who exploited me for the doctor's own professional gain, personal self-interests, and financial profits and who was clearly not qualified to cosmetically work on me, having had multiple cosmetic surgeries. I wish I had only done my homework before embarking on finding the right cosmetic or plastic surgeon for myself. I wish I had found a Certified American Board Plastic Surgeon, who could do what I cosmetically wanted, needed, and expected of him—or simply leave my nose and ears just the way he found them when I initially walked into the doctor's office. I wish the reader all the best in finding the right cosmetic or plastic surgeon for himself or herself.

I make an appeal to the reader to urge your legislators, congressmen and women, judges and courts, and medical boards to put a stop to all medical malpractice crimes, exploitation, and abuses by changing the laws of the medical boards to make certain that they have a criminal enforcement team in each Medical Quality Assurance Commission in Victimized, USA. I recognize that we can make a difference in the battle against medical malpractice victimization if we let our voices be heard that we will no longer tolerate medical malpractice victimization in our United States or in any other country in the world.

Dr. Cutter eventually moved out of Victimized, USA, to Victimization, USA. Other people call it Lake Placid, USA.

I believe my personal complaint played a role in Dr. Cutter's decision to move to another region.

This book is written with the long-range goal that no longer will the trusting public be victimized by those in positions of trust. Medical malpractice acts caused by medical doctors must be stopped.

May the victimization of Kurtess Scone, and other unsuspecting cosmetic consumers be immediately put to an end. May the malicious actions of all medical doctors never get to be repeated on any innocent, unsuspecting person ever again. I would like for every citizen in Victimized, USA, to make an urgent appeal to his or her congressmen to pass a law stating that once a medical board or dental board complaint is submitted or reported to the police, medical boards, legislators, or insurance companies, the statute of limitations immediately is extended for the lifetime of the victimized patient. I hope there will no longer be a three- or four-year statute of limitations ruling for every victimized consumer.

I sincerely would like to thank everyone who can identify with what I have painfully experienced. I only hope that there will be many who have been encouraged, inspired, and motivated to take action to help put an end to all forms of hurtful and destructive victimization as a positive consequence of reading my book.

Read on for my advice to all.

ADVICE TO THE READER

I offer some good advice for my readers to benefit from. If you or someone you know has been victimized, used, or misused by a medical doctor, please pray for those who have physically harmed you.

Jesus tells us in St. Matthew's gospel to pray for those who spitefully use us. That would include a medical doctor using you in a mean, cruel, or malicious way for professional gain and personal profit.

Keep in mind that God says, "Beloved, do not avenge yourselves, but rather give place to wrath; for it is written, 'Vengeance is Mine, I will repay,' says the Lord" (Rom. 12:19, NKJV).

You might say, "But I'm not a Christian nor a believer in Jesus Christ, so what am I supposed to do with my angry, vengeful, and bitter feelings toward those who have harmed me in this case?"

I recommend that you never give up on yourself, but take your hurt feelings and try to go through the motions of surrendering them up to God anyway. Although you don't believe in Him, this practice is still a healthy way to free yourself from becoming a bitter, critical, discouraged, and a depressing kind of person to be around. God will lovingly accept your efforts to free yourself from painful feelings you experienced needlessly at the hands of a person you trusted. If you can only believe with a small measure of faith in a great big loving God, He will absorb your pain as your shock absorber. Be an encourager to others; do not be a discourager in life. Be part of the solution in this negative world, and not part of the problem. Holding on to negative feelings is destructive to one's mental, emotional, and physical well-being.

Remember your goals in life. You should report any doctor that caused you great physical pain in any way, shape, or form to the Better Business Bureau, the Attorney General, and the medical boards and commissions they may be licensed with; and if you know that a crime has taken place, feel perfectly free to contact legal authorities and report the crime that has taken place against yourself or someone you know.

There were many other things that I did during the course of my life—so many that if they were all written down, it would require that another book be written or that the current book be much longer.

The events recorded in this book, *The Ultimate Violation,* are to equip the reader to avoid the wrong doctors and the major pitfalls that I fell into in my search for the right cosmetic or plastic surgeon for myself. Hopefully, you will now be able to find the right medical doctor, who will be a good, honest, and truthful communicator. He or she will be a medical doctor who rightly interprets exactly what you may want, need, and expect from your surgery procedure, and has the medical specialties skills that provide the best-quality cosmetic results. Best wishes in finding the right cosmetic or plastic surgeon who can meet your cosmetic needs to your satisfaction.

Sincerely,
Kurtess Leif Scone

Postscript: To-Do List

I have provided a checklist for the reader to fill out in order to prevent ever being victimized by a medical doctor in your search for the right cosmetic or plastic surgeon for your cosmetic interests:

1. Make certain the medical doctor is a Certified American Board Plastic Surgeon and has done a great number of the same procedures you want to have done.
2. Make certain the cosmetic surgeon is listed with the American Board of Medical Specialties (ABMS), which is considered a recognized board.
3. Have the medical doctor explain in detail what he is planning to do to your physical characteristics or body part. Make sure that explanation clearly matches up with your cosmetic or reconstructive interests.
4. Inquire if you could have a friend or family member videotape your consultations with the cosmetic or plastic surgeon.
5. Make sure you have a friend or family member with you during your consultations.
6. Find out what kind of training the doctor has received to cosmetically perform surgical procedures with precision skill on your physical features or body part.
7. Ask for names of patients who have had cosmetic surgery by this doctor on the same body part with similar presurgery conditions as you.
8. Make certain that you have done your homework before embarking on your search for the right cosmetic or plastic surgeon for yourself.
9. Request any complaints that have been filed against the medical doctor with the health department and medical boards he or she is licensed in your state.
10. Have the friend or family member who provided the ride for you remain with you until you are on the surgery table and have been prepared for surgery. You may even request to have them stay with you

during surgery to be a witness for any last-minute changes the surgeon may state out loud in front of his assistants or whisper to the patient before you go under local or general anesthesia.

11. Have a good attorney selected prior to surgery should the surgeon change plans on you on the day of surgery that in any way leave you mentally dazed, confused, and perplexed pre- or postsurgery.

12. Inquire what the doctor's qualifications are to perform the cosmetic procedure on your physical characteristics or body part with precision skill.

13. Inquire what the medical doctor's specialty is versus what his or her subspecialties are.

14. Feel free to ask a lot of questions of the medical doctor because your future happiness, mental sanity, and peace of mind depend on your whole person being satisfied that you were not used, abused, and victimized for the medical doctor's professional gain and personal profit.

15. Don't be concerned with thinking you're going to embarrass yourself by asking too many questions relevant to your cosmetic interests.

16. Should you find a medical doctor who hedges, hesitates, or refuses to communicate with you to your satisfaction, feel perfectly free to not pursue a cosmetic relationship with the medical doctor; should you be in the cosmetic surgeon's presence, request to leave the doctor's office immediately with haste.

FOOD FOR THOUGHT

In life there are those who make things happen, those who watch things happen, and then those who wonder what did happen. Perhaps you see yourself falling into one of these categories. Perhaps you have a natural curiosity about how any person could ever be victimized by a cosmetic surgeon disguised as a caring medical doctor. Perhaps you are interested in watching and reading about criminal cases and the mystery of how the police end up solving the cases.

I never had a brother named Steven S. Scone, but let's imagine I did. Steven would have taught the good, uncaring doctor a lesson on the doctor's nose and ears as payback when the medical doctor said to me, "It didn't turn out as I envisioned." Steven would have said to the doctor, "Let's see if this turns out as I envision."

Steven would then have introduced the doctor to flying lessons—into the wall and then onto the floor. Steven Scone would have had a session of private hands-on counseling with Dr. Cutter. Dr. Cutter not only would have learned how to fly, but he would also have learned some new dance steps.

The above scenario is totally fictitious because I never had a brother named Steven S. Scone. I wrote this book with the earnest hope that patient victimization will become a thing of the past. The above fictitious character named Steven was only reenacted as a fantasy role played out as an event as food for thought to the reader.

My wish is that all who have read this book will come to the knowledge of God and will openly accept Jesus, who is the only One that can truly help us through any circumstance we encounter.